"*In my years as practicing physician, author and editor, I have never met anyone more capable or more dedicated than Rajgopal Nidamboor, especially in the field of mind-body/integrative medicine*".

-Dr Richard Firshein, Director, Firshein Center for Comprehensive Medicine, and author of Reversing Asthma and The Nutraceutical Revolution, New York, US.

CONTENTS

CONTENTS

CONTENTS

CONTENTS

INTRODUCTION

The most common form of joint affection, osteoarthritis [OA] is a degenerative disorder. It affects millions of people worldwide — it's seemingly more common than heart disease and diabetes.

Call it a paradox, or what you may, one major fact remains: osteoarthritis is only going to expand in its intensity, and also get firmly rooted in one's middle years, sooner rather than later. Experts estimate that it may afflict over 250 million worldwide in the next fifteen years. In the UK, experts estimate that over three million people visit their doctor for osteoarthritis, every year.

There is no easy answer, much less a cure for osteoarthritis. Forget about lasting relief. The rationale? Conventional medicine has nothing much to offer, much less to repair, or rebuild, an osteoarthritic joint. What's more, most prescription medicines have a host of side-effects, even if they "ease" the symptoms of osteoarthritic pain. This isn't all. NSAIDs [non-steroidal anti-inflammatory drugs], for instance, offer relief from pain, all right — but, they are evidenced to cause and/or promote serious side-effects.

NSAIDs are a large group of medications used to treat pain and inflammation [response of the immune system to infection]. There are several types of NSAIDs, aspirin, being the most common. Other examples of NSAIDs are ibuprofen, naproxen, piroxicam and nabumetone.

Despite their clear efficacy in the management of inflammation, the very "hub" of arthritic pain, NSAIDs are a significant cause and concern for adverse events, particularly gastro-intestinal ulceration/bleeding and compromised kidney function. Which, inevitably, leads us to one big question — is there a way out of this "complexity," even if osteoarthritis is not life-threatening; or quite disabling, if left untreated and unattended?

Yes — there is hope. In the form of natural dietary supplements, or natural "nutrients," glucosamine and chondroitin — at a time when conventional medicine is grossly restricted in its ability to merely address symptoms of osteoarthritis. It does not help you get over it — lock, stock and barrel.

The two "nutraceuticals" — glucosamine and chondroitin — are more than useful and dependable in managing OA. Nutraceuticals are phytochemicals, or functional foods; they are natural, bioactive chemical compounds that have health-promoting, disease-preventing, and medicinal properties. In addition to reversing the damage caused by osteoarthritis, glucosamine and chondroitin also get to the "root" of the problem, and revamp joint cartilage.

What's more, researchers have, over the past decade, made exciting strides discovering that dietary supplementation with cartilage, or its key chemical components — glucosamine and chondroitin — can help protect and/or even restore damaged cartilage. They also contend that the two nutraceutical supplements enhance the feeling of well-being, mainly because your joints are growing [a]new. Next, they infer, that the duo restores the cushioning between the spaces, where bones meet, with healthy cartilage.

However, cautious optimism is necessary. The two, separately, or in combination, do not hold the magic wand to blow your symptoms, or problems, away. What they actually do is give palpable relief from pain, and also reduce the difficulty of movement common in osteoarthritic patients.

Think all this sounds exaggerated — or, well-orchestrated hard sell or hoopla? The fact is: scientifically-based clinical trials offer a dependable grounding in favour of glucosamine and chondroitin in real pain relief for osteoarthritic joints — a long-term treatment plan you'd call upon and trust.

This handy book brings to you responsible information on glucosamine and chondroitin, based on scientific analysis. It takes a realistic view of other treatment options too, including the role of conventional medications, alternative remedies, and additional supplements.

Finally, what you will also get to know is not a panacea, but a realistic, workable plan based on safety, and well-being, with minimum risks and/or side-effects.

Isn't this reason enough for you to give glucosamine and chondroitin a real, good chance to "engineer" a truly safe, welcome break from pain for your ailing joints? Read on...

****

Chapter 1

HOW JOINTS WORK

First, the basics. A joint is the point where two bones meet. The human body has more than one hundred joints. These joints make up what is referred to as the articular system; they are also responsible for body movements.

The co-operative manoeuvre of three kinds of joints is responsible for different motion capabilities, viz., cartilaginous, fibrous, and synovial. The joints between the ribs, that are slightly movable, are cartilaginous in nature; the bones of the skull, not generally movable, are fibrous in form; and, joints such as the elbow, fingers, hips, and knees, the most complex and endowed with maximum movements, make up the synovial joints. These joints contain what is called the synovial fluid — a sticky fluid, or natural lubricant, that provides the joints with the ease of movement, which we often take for granted.

Synovial fluid is produced in the synovial membrane, which lines the joint; it supplies the building blocks for the repair of cartilage and also removes waste products. The fluid is vital for healthy joints, mainly because cartilage is not endowed with its own blood supply chain.

Our joints, in effect, are excellent biomechanical systems whose health and vitality are regulated by a highly advanced, or sophisticated, chemical feedback loop. This makes our joints not only complex, but also vulnerable — because, a problem in any part of the joint can cause a domino effect that can throw the entire system out of gear. As we age, our body's amazing structure which gives our joints *that* remarkable flexibility seems to lose its knack of absorbing stress as we do without difficulty when we're younger. So, once the balance is disturbed, we have the following unwelcome portrait to contend with:

- Cartilage will deteriorate; it may also develop ulcers; the synovial fluid leaks into the subchondral bone [bone to which cartilage is attached], causing cysts in the marrow
- The subchondral bone may develop minuscule fractures and rough spurs [bony projections]; they also form calluses [thick, hardened, dead skin], and solidify
- Synovial cells may form tiny pellets of bone and connective tissue called osteophytes — these collect in the synovial fluid and cause further damage
- The synovial membranes thicken, and this reduces the joint space
- As the disease progresses into "full-blown" osteoarthritis, inflammation may now occur in the synovial membrane, causing chondrocytes [cartilage cells] to manufacture the wrong type of collagen — a classical case of a marvellously organised biochemical system gone *kaput.*

THE TROUBLE WITH OSTEOARTHRITIS

A bone-joint disorder, and not as significantly inflammatory in nature, or form, as rheumatoid arthritis [RA], a related disorder, osteoarthritis — or, what is also called *osteoarthrosis* — has a definitive affinity to affect the highly movable synovial joints.

It is not that cartilaginous joints are exempt; however, osteoarthritis is relatively uncommon in them. As a matter of fact, the term, osteoarthrosis, mirrors the nature of the disorder, whose basic cause of pain is related to the gradual decay of cartilage and subchondral bone.

Osteoarthritis, to put it mildly, robs you of your basic ability to get fully engaged in day-to-day activity. When it escalates, it may confine you to your bed — even for days at a stretch. In its early stages, it may affect one joint, or multiple joints; besides, it may vary in its intensity, or severity. The result: one may experience mild pain and stiffness and/or crippling aches, aside from joint deformity.

Needless to say, osteoarthritis is one of man's oldest afflictions. By way of medical definition, it is a chronic disease that involves the breakdown of joints and surrounding tissue. The name is derived from the Greek: "osteo," refers to bones; "orthro," to joints involved; and, "itis," to the inflammatory process of the disease. In simple terms, osteoarthritis is a typical progression of events "prompted" by normal aging, physical injury, chronic joint stress, oxidative stress, and genetic anomalies.

It's all in the gut is not just a literary metaphor. It may be a pointer, or *raison d'être*, for osteoarthritis to surface — more so, when your gut is not in good health, or shape.

The problem in osteoarthritis essentially lies with the cartilage — the natural cushion that protects the ends of bones. Complaints related to the disease emerge as the bones grind together, owing to what was once erroneously referred to as "wear and tear," due to aging.

The understanding today is osteoarthritis is caused when the body's healthy cartilage is unable to function at its optimum level and/or efficiency.

Briefly...

> - Osteoarthritis is inflammation of the joints; it results from cartilage degeneration
> - It can be caused by aging, heredity, and injury from trauma or disease
> - The most common symptom is pain in the affected joint/s after repetitive use
> - There is no specific blood test for the diagnosis of the disorder
> - The objective of treatment in osteoarthritis is to reduce joint pain and inflammation, while improving and maintaining joint function.

IT'S ALL IN THE CARTILAGE

The building block of bone, skin, tendon, and other connective tissues, the cartilage not only provides tissue cushioning to the ends of bones where the joints meet, but it also allows for flexible movement. You may call cartilage nature's own shock absorbers.

Cartilage encompasses three basic substances: a special kind of protein called collagen, a compound made of protein and sugar called proteoglycans, and water, which gives it resiliency. Collagen fibres form the matrix of cartilage, just as much as proteoglycans perform the mop-like effect to trap water within the [cartilage] structure. The water, thus "engulfed," allows the cartilage to absorb shock and spring back after being compressed during what may, in effect, be referred to as normal movement.

In addition to this, our cartilage also contains cells called chondrocytes. Chondrocytes are responsible for the manufacture of new collagen and proteoglycans. They also secrete enzymes to "wipe out" old collagen and proteoglycans molecules. More of this later.

When chondrocytes malfunction, it disturbs the balance between the degraded enzymes and the rebuilding process. In addition to this, the proteoglycans that emerge from a malfunctioning chondrocyte are often incomplete and defective; they are not up to the task of providing strong cartilage. Result: the right type of "soil" is set for the onset of osteoarthritis.

Put simply, the awesome threesome, described in the preceding paragraph, offers our body the means to absorb "shock" from daily activity — be it walking, running, jumping, and so on.

For one who is overweight, it is easy to guess how the weight-bearing joints need to sustain pressure during active use. The more the weight, the more the burden.

Generally speaking, nature has endowed us with the ability to absorb shocks and pressure, but when our joints are affected by osteoarthritis, regular activities can be a nightmare — a great "invite" to pain.

Briefly...

> **Cartilage is made up of four substances: collagen, proteoglycans, water and chondrocytes**
> - *Collagen.* A key component of cartilage, collagen provides cartilage with strength. It creates the framework to accommodate other components of cartilage
> - *Proteoglycans.* A combination of protein and sugar, proteoglycan[s] is woven around and through collagen. This allows the cartilage to change shape when
>   compressed. Proteoglycans also trap water in cartilage, which is reallocated with movement

- *Water.* Healthy cartilage contains more than 70 per cent water. Water absorbs shock in the cartilage; it also lubricates and nourishes the cartilage
- *Chondrocytes.* These cells produce new collagen and proteoglycans in cartilage. They also release enzymes, which help break down and dispose of aging collagen and proteoglycans.

CAUSES OF OSTEOARTHRITIS

Age

The risk of osteoarthritis increases with age. However, after the age of 70, the risk drops down, mainly due to a decrease in heavy physical activity.

Gender

After the age of 55-60, women have a higher incidence of osteoarthritis of the knee than do men. Some studies suggest that the decline in native oestrogen after menopause may play a role in amplified OA risk in women, since oestrogen replacement therapy is primarily associated with reduced risk.

Women with generalised osteoarthritis [hands, spine, knees and/or hips] appear to have a marginally increased risk of premature death too.

Obesity

Studies have suggested the risk of osteoarthritis of the knee joint in women increased 40 per cent for each 10-pound weight gain. A body of medical opinion insists that if obesity were eliminated, the incidence of osteoarthritis of the knee joint in both men and women would fall by 25-50 per cent.

Previous injury

Joint injury, such as a tear in the knee, increases the risk of osteoarthritis. Osteoarthritis occurs more rapidly in older adults with joint injuries than in younger people. Individuals who have held, or hold, jobs requiring intense physical labour repeatedly "endure" chronic joint damage. This often leads to osteoarthritis.

Muscle weakness

Studies have shown that weakness in the quadriceps muscle [the muscle that runs from the front of the thigh across the knee, and down to the shin] is associated with osteoarthritis of the knee in people over age 65. Besides, a decline in the strength of the knee, with age, also leads to increased risk of osteoarthritis.

Congenital abnormalities

A structural abnormality, like congenital hip dysplasia [a childhood condition caused by abnormal development of the hip joint], can lead to osteoarthritis in later life, mainly due to changes in the shape of the joint.

Joint infections

Though this is uncommon, joints can be infected by bacteria, viruses, fungi, and mycobacteria [organisms that cause tuberculosis]. They can infiltrate the joint spaces. Outcome: acute and chronic damage, in the long run, and also impending osteoarthritis. Some of the most infamous microbes that infect the joints include the bacteria that also cause Lyme disease [a bacterial disorder] and gonorrhoea.

Metabolic and hormonal disturbances

A host of disorders characterises osteoarthritis as a complication. They include Paget's disease [in which the bones are remodelled inappropriately], acromegaly [a slow progressive disease characterised by excessive circulating growth hormone], and haemochromatosis [iron storage disease].

Diet

Recent studies have shown that high levels of vitamin C and vitamin D in the diet may be beneficial in osteoarthritis. In one study, evidence of continuing joint damage was reduced three-fold in people with the highest dietary intake of vitamins C and D.

****

Chapter 2

TYPES OF OSTEOARTHRITIS

There are two types of osteoarthritis.

Primary osteoarthritis is the more common form of osteoarthritis. Its exact cause is not known. Some experts believe that both obesity and family history of the disease may have a say in its onset. Slow, or insidious, in origin, it often affects the knees and the hips.

Secondary osteoarthritis, the other form, is, generally, attributed to a specific cause — a traumatic event, such as an accident, or sports injury.

Other causes include joint infection, surgery of the joint and/or chronic trauma caused due to recurrent, or repetitive, movement — for example, sport activity — that damages the joint, metabolic imbalance in the form of calcium deposits, or chronic overuse of a joint, especially from hard labour. In other words, any activity that calls for sustained overuse of the joints can lead to secondary osteoarthritis.

Needless to say, secondary osteoarthritis is common in the younger population. However, this does not mean that regular exercise can lead to osteoarthritis. Just the opposite. Regular physical activity can help reduce "the kick in the joint," if not the "teeth," of osteoarthritis.

All the same, the best way to prevent osteoarthritis is by way of recalling a Shakespearean aphorism: "The better part of valour is discretion." This should also offer an objective lesson to those engaged in extended physical activity, or sport. The watchword? Play by all means; but, also take care of your joints.

WHAT HAPPENS ACTUALLY

The first thing that takes place when a joint is affected by osteoarthritis is a "boom" in the enzymes that break down proteoglycans. Add to this new proteoglycans that cannot just cope with the destruction, and you have collagen fibres that become totally exposed to enzymes. So, you have an obvious pattern in the final stages of osteoarthritis: the entire cartilage matrix being dissolved, as it were. In addition, the chondrocytes now "wane" and the ends of bones are unduly pushed into rubbing painfully together. As our body's defence mechanism now comes in to protect the joint from the "invasion," the area affected becomes inflamed. This leads to the breakdown of tissue and extended pain in the affected joint.

WHO'S WHO OF OA

We all know of an obvious paradox. Age has something to do with wisdom — and, vice versa. Or, osteoarthritis? The joint disease generally sets in around 40; and, its risk increases dramatically with age. The incidence of osteoarthritis seems to be growing by two per cent each year in the United States alone and nearly fifty per cent of Americans in the age group of 65+ are afflicted with the disease.

This is not all. Since the number of older people is also increasing, so too is the incidence of osteoarthritis worldwide. However, for one who's below the age of 40, the beginning is quite often related to a specific joint injury.

The disease affects both men and women equally — the difference being of degree. Men often develop osteoarthritis before age 45; for women, it is often after age 45. Besides, if a close family member has osteoarthritis, the chances of your getting it are greater. Not only that. Obesity is another precursor of osteoarthritis — thanks to the "song of the burden" of extra weight your joints have to contend with.

It is not, however, exactly known why obesity increases the risk of osteoarthritis. What is quite well known is weight loss can keep the disease at bay — and, this is good enough reason for us to maintain our weight on a scale that suits us best.

SYMPTOM PICTURE

Remember the time when you first felt your joint — especially, your knee — was a wee bit stiff in the morning? You gobbled up a pill, or did nothing. May be, you'd also remember that the pain was irregular; perhaps, with one side of the body involved. You'd also recall that this began to change, down the line, and you experienced pain in multiple joints. You also had to put up with pain anytime and/or throughout the day, when activity of any form was initiated.

You felt better with rest, and as the disease began to get entrenched bit by bit, you experienced pain with the most trivial of movements — even at rest.

Briefly...

Symptoms of Osteoarthritis

- Pain, commonly in the hands, knee, and hip joints; sometimes in the spine
- Pain often related to activity of the joint; pain, generally worse at the end of the day and/or after periods of activity [As the disease advances in its intensity, pain is also present during rest]
- Stiffness, following long periods of inactivity, especially in the morning after a goodnight's sleep and/or after sitting for a long time

---

- Restricted movement of the joint
- Tenderness [sensitivity] and occasional swelling
- Deformity of the joints — most notably seen when the disease progresses to its crescendo
- Cracking of the joints, accompanied by pain [This may also occur in a normal joint, not affected by osteoarthritis. It is usually painless].

REFERRED PAIN

A progressive disease, osteoarthritis tends to worsen over a period of time. In the most advanced cases, bones can get deformed just as much as bone spurs [projections] are formed. Shooting pains down the arms and back of the thighs are also as common as pain up the back of the head. These are often called "referred pain." One may also experience "cracking" in the joints — with a distinct audible sound and/or a sensation of crunching. Not a painful experience by any means at least initially, the sound can sometimes be loud — and, that's about it. But, it could burrow a corridor of uncertainty in one's mind.

True inflammation is not often a primary symptom in osteoarthritis. It is a late entrant — quite unlike the intensity that is characteristic of rheumatoid arthritis [RA], an auto-immune disorder, and a different form of the disease.

Briefly...

A variety of factors can increase your risk of developing osteoarthritis. Here they are, in précis:

Age	Age is the strongest risk factor for osteoarthritis. It can appear in young adulthood. You are at higher risk, if you're over 45. The risk increases after age 65
Gender	The disorder is more common in women than in men
Heredity	People born with defective cartilage, or with joints that don't fit together appropriately, are more likely to develop osteoarthritis
Joint injury or overuse	Traumatic injury to the knee or hip increases your risk of developing osteoarthritis. Also, joints that are used repeatedly in certain occupations, or sports, may more likely develop osteoarthritis due to injury and/or overuse
Overweight	Carrying excess weight during, or after midlife, is a significant risk factor for osteoarthritis of the knee joint.

****

Chapter 3

DIAGNOSIS

The most obvious symptom of osteoarthritis is, of course, joint pain during or after use. In severe cases, your joints will ache even when you are inactive. You may also experience stiffness and swelling in your joints, especially when you wake up in the morning. This stiffness generally fades away in less than half-an-hour.

Osteoarthritis doesn't always announce itself. In fact, many people with osteoarthritis of the fingers don't even know they have the condition, even if X-rays clearly show deteriorating cartilage in their joints.

Osteoarthritis in the knees and hips, however, usually causes significant pain. Women with osteoarthritis of the hands, for example, often develop bony lumps at the ends of their fingers. These are called Heberden's nodes. The lumps are not common in men; they may be painful to begin with, and one often tends to think of them as a cosmetic glitch. But, the fact is: osteoarthritis is a permanent condition, even if the nagging pain eases in its intensity over time.

Diagnosing osteoarthritis is not as easy as you'd think. There is no one sure-fire test. What is often recommended is a combination of methods — to rule out other conditions that mimic the ailment.

Your physician/therapist may ask you a set of questions mainly to determine the clinical history of the onset of the disease — especially in reference to pain, stiffness, and limitations, if any, in the affected joint. A physical examination is done next to evaluate how restricted the joint use actually is.

Briefly...

X-Rays
X-rays of the bones and joints in an osteoarthritic individual will show narrowing of the spaces that should be seen in joints. Also indicative of the disease are thickening of the bone that lines the joints, besides the formation of bone spurs. X-rays may also show possible bone changes, indicative of osteoarthritis — and, this will include individuals who report none of the common symptoms of the disease.

MRI
MRI [Magnetic Resonance Imaging] studies are very sensitive tests. They are, in the main, used to diagnose acute injuries; they can also help detect early signs of osteoarthritis before classical symptoms are manifest.

Ultrasound
Ultrasounds of osteoarthritic joints are particularly good at finding effusions [fluid collection] that might be too small to produce an obvious swelling. However, despite the sensitivity of ultrasound and MRI, most radiologists prefer the use of X-ray as being enough to arrive at a diagnosis.

X-rays are usually used to measure the extent of joint damage, but they do not match with the intensity of the pain, or extent of disability in the individual. While X-rays can provide key information on the quantum of cartilage loss, bone damage, or bone spurs, they may not provide a clear clue, as some authorities deduce, to detecting osteoarthritis early.

Confirmation of osteoarthritis is done by extracting some fluid from the affected joint and examining it microscopically — for the presence of micro-organisms, uric acid, and other substances. Culture studies of the sample are also undertaken to analyse for other infections, just as much as blood tests are used to determine the presence of proteins characteristic of rheumatoid arthritis [RA], or elevated levels of uric acid common to gout [a metabolic disorder of the big toe].

Your doctor will also use tests to rule out other joint disorders, including bursitis [inflammation of a bursa, a sac-like membrane, between bone and tissue, near a joint], which often imitates symptoms of osteoarthritis. In addition, you could undergo arthroscopy, a surgical technique, in which a specialist inserts a viewing tube into the joint space.

Once a diagnosis is confirmed, the next step for you is to determine what would be most ideally suited to regain, or help restore, your quality of life to the maximum extent possible.

Enter, glucosamine and chondroitin — and, you have the right answer — to reduce and alleviate your osteoarthritic agony.

WHY GLUCOSAMINE AND CHONDROITIN?

Simple. Glucosamine is a natural product found in our body. It helps build and maintain cartilage, tendons and other connective tissues of the body, while inhibiting the growth of cartilage-destroying enzymes — the main shock absorber of our body. Besides, there is another plus — clinical trials have reported more side-effects caused by a sugar-covered placebo [dummy pill] than by glucosamine, not to mention some major side-effects of NSAIDs!

This is not all. While glucosamine plays a key role in cartilage formation and repair, chondroitin is part of a large protein molecule [proteoglycans] that gives cartilage its elasticity.

Glucosamine also prevents other body enzymes from degrading the building blocks of joint cartilage. In addition, glucosamine and chondroitin can relieve joint pain, and actually help rebuild cartilage, while slowing down the progression of osteoarthritis.

What does this signify? That glucosamine and chondroitin are the basic building blocks for proteoglycans; they also appear to stimulate chondrocytes to make new collagen and proteoglycans. In addition to this, anecdotal evidence from millions of glucosamine/chondroitin users reporting pain relief and the ability to take part in activities that were all too painful, or difficult, earlier, has also been followed by scientific studies. This also demonstrates the fact that glucosamine and chondroitin provide a natural "boost" to joint health. Also, new research has shown that oral supplementation of proteoglycans precursors, like the two supplements, leads to articular cartilage repair.

The inference? Glucosamine and chondroitin significantly reduce joint pain and stiffness; this relief is better than or equal to ibuprofen, for example, but without the latter's dangerous side-effects. There is also evidence that glucosamine maintains our joint space while increasing function and flexibility.

Glucosamine and chondroitin are both components of normal cartilage; they are available in pharmacies and health food stores, as nutritional supplements, without a prescription. The supplements are well tolerated and safe. And, because the duo stimulates the production of new cartilage components, experts suggest that they are able to help the body repair damaged cartilage.

This is good enough reason to try them — and, derive benefits. Naturally. Right? You bet.

DEFECT AND EFFECT

More than a handful of theories are doing the rounds in the causative process of osteoarthritis. One of them relates to the fact that what goes haywire in the cartilage repair process can lead to osteoarthritis. Another holds on to the view that chondrocytes that make new cartilage may have "cooked" the wrong mixture of ingredients, just as much as they are packing too many of the cartilage-destroyer enzymes, but not adequate materials needed to build new cartilage.

Further, for a long time it was thought that chondrocytes' malfunction was not a reversible process. Research, in the recent past, united by a host of scientific studies, has shown that this isn't quite the case. The inference is obvious. Glucosamine and chondroitin have it in them to provide the gentle push your body needs to not only correct, but also rectify the snags that occur in the body's process of creating new, healthy cartilage.

PREVENTING OA

While osteoarthritis may not be a completely curable disease, it is not really a predestined product of the aging process. Like any problem that ought to have solution, osteoarthritis is a disease you can ward off for as long as may be possible.

While the most important preventive tool is the good, age-old, or time-proven exercise, avoiding injuries is another vital component of any prevention plan. There is, of course, no foolproof method to avoiding injuries, but it is within our grasp to minimising risks.
Here are some useful examples: correct footwear; a proper ergonomic chair for those who sit for long periods; and, appropriate

posture. Also, it is best to protect your joints from serious injury or repeated minor injuries. This will decrease your risk of damaging your cartilage, more so because repeated minor injuries including job-related injuries, such as frequent or constant kneeling, squatting, or other postures, place stress and strain on the knee joint.

Exercise is the best recipe for osteoarthritis, thanks to the unique anatomy of our joints. Joints don't have blood supply to nourish them, unlike other body tissues. They obtain oxygen and nourishment; they eliminate waste as a result of movement. So, the equation is simple: without joint activity and motion, our joints get depleted of oxygen and other nutrients. This leads to joint degeneration and osteoarthritis.

Exercise can often help reduce joint pain and stiffness. Light to moderate physical activity may prevent problems setting in; they may also restore health and function. However, the fact remains: some people with osteoarthritis may be reluctant to exercise because of joint pain after activity. Various steps can be taken to help relieve pain, such as heat and cold therapy or natural pain relievers [ginger, or turmeric], which may make it easier for you to exercise and stay active. The most recommended method is partial or non-weight bearing exercise — viz., cycling, swimming, yoga, or aquatic exercises.

Yet another key element is weight control. Maintaining a healthy and appropriate weight may be the single most important thing one can do to prevent osteoarthritis. If losing unhealthy weight to prevent, or lessen, joint damage and decrease the stress on osteoarthritic joints is ideal, being overweight places extra strain on the joints, particularly the large weight-bearing joints, such as the knees, the hips, and the balls of the feet. Aside from this, extra weight may also alter the normal structure of the joint and increase the risk of osteoarthritis.

Maintaining a healthy weight is, therefore, ideal. This may help to reduce the risk of osteoarthritis, because the strain on the weight-bearing joints, if one is on the unhealthy side of the weight index, can, in the long run, destroy the joint.

Experts also suggest that overweight men and women are 30 per cent more likely than their normal weight counterparts to develop osteoarthritis. The more the weight, the worse it is. As a matter of fact, obese men and women have a higher risk percentage [ratio of 70:50] in developing osteoarthritis. What is, for that reason, good news to your joints is losing weight and maintaining it at a level that keeps the osteoarthritic "wolf" from your body's, nay joint's, door.

Researchers also reckon that the decay of proteoglycans is central to the disease process in a majority of osteoarthritic cases. As we age, our proteoglycans tend to become small[er] and "tap" less water around themselves — this is, in effect, due to the smaller size of chondroitin sulphate chains. More of this later. Also, infection, or inflammation, can often produce abnormal amounts of free radicals. This leads to degradation of cartilage tissue and, at the same time, stimulates the release of cartilage-dissolving enzymes, thanks to decreased chondroitin sulphate, a favoured nutraceutical supplement. Add to this, a poor anti-oxidant diet in any population, and this leaves our tissues open to free radical damage.
Now, you have the rationale why aging, damaged, and malnourished cartilage, needs anti-oxidants like vitamin C to neutralise free radicals, along with a regular supply of glucosamine/chondroitin sulphate to repair and also generate proteoglycans. If this is not done, our cartilage will begin to fall to pieces, like a pack of cards.

Other measures

Calcium is indispensable for optimal bone health. Researchers explain that weak bones can increase the progression of osteoarthritis. Nutritionists recommend 4-5 servings of low-fat dairy products, per day, to get your calcium requirement. If you don't fancy the idea, you'd try other fortified foods and/or supplements available in the market. In addition, it would be advisable for you to —

- Keep a close watch on your posture. Proper posture can help reduce and prevent osteoarthritis pain, especially in your back, hips, and knees

- Accept and begin to live with the problem; develop a positive attitude. If you have arthritis in your fingers, you may opt for shoes that fasten with Velcro; not laces. Simple idea; but it could offer you comfort and confidence

- Get in touch with a support group in your area. It helps — psychologically. It is a well-known fact that sharing your experiences, with others, can be profoundly comforting. Most support groups offer you practical tips for coping with osteoarthritis.

****

Chapter 4

HEALING THROUGH DESIGN

Any effective treatment plan for osteoarthritis is related to address two main objectives. The first objective is to control pain *per se*; the second to slow down, and, if possible, reverse the progression of the disease.

But, one fact remains: conventional treatment today offers quite a handful of remedial measures, and more, in the treatment of osteoarthritis. However, in reality, it provides just symptomatic relief, not viable, long-term respite. Conventional treatment, at best, may be referred to as palliative, not all-encompassing. Besides this, you have the spectre of a "grand" side-effect profile of such medicines used.

Glucosamine and chondroitin meet the basic parameters in the osteoarthritis treatment plan. They offer both pain relief and control. In addition, they provide recovery of cartilage function and promote healing — all without the flagrant side-effects of conventional medications. Also, the two supplements extend sustained comfort from joint pain and tenderness [sensitivity to touch] and, in the process, improve mobility. Naturally. Safely.

GLUCOSAMINE

Glucosamine [pronounced, *glue-koe-sah-meen*] is the basic building block for proteoglycans. Proteoglycans, as described earlier, act like sponge to retain water so essential for vibrant joint function.

In simple terms, glucose, or sugar, and an amino acid, or protein building block, are combined to form glucosamine. Nature has endowed our body to manufacture its own glucosamine. However, in osteoarthritis an extra amount of glucosamine supply can bring about a world of difference to joint health.

The reason is simple. Glucosamine helps make cartilage in joints; it is also needed for the formation of blood vessels, bone, ligaments, nails, skin, synovial fluid, and tendons, aside from mucous secretions of our digestive tract. More importantly, glucosamine is fundamentally needed by our body to make chondroitin.

Taken orally in capsule or tablet form, glucosamine is absorbed from the gastro-intestinal [GI] tract quickly and almost fully [approximately 90 per cent]. Once absorbed, the body sends a bulk of the "wrapped up" compound to areas of cartilage — to build new and healthy cartilage.

The growing interest worldwide in glucosamine and chondroitin is not new. As already mentioned, glucosamine is a substance naturally occurring in our body. That it was synthesised more than 100 years ago may be news to most of us; what may also be news is researchers got the first clue, in the mid-1950s. That the substance could play an active role in the treatment of osteoarthritis.

The first uncontrolled studies were, of course, not meticulous — if not totally flawed. They also invited scepticism for "positive" results — as a result of "fanciful" thinking by both physicians/therapist and their patients — when no conclusive proof was verifiable.

The idea may not have changed very much today, although several research studies in many countries, aside from the US, have showed that glucosamine really helps joint. This has spawned the New Collagen Era. What's more, it has also given enough impetus for further studies.

A bit of narration, again. By the end of the 1960s, glucosamine was documented to relieve patients affected by osteoarthritis. However, it was only recently that researchers began to develop a more stable and dependable compound with a long shelf-life.

In the early days, glucosamine was injected to bring about relief from pain and improve mobility in patients. It was difficult and cumbersome.

In the course of time, glucosamine became available in an oral pill/tablet form; this is, obviously, a much-preferred choice like any other medication, today.

CHONDROITIN

Chondroitin [pronounced, *kon-droy-tin*], or chondroitin sulphate, to use its technical name, is quite like glucosamine. It is made within the body. It is also an essential component of cartilage and other connective tissues. It belongs to a group of compounds called Glycosaminoglycans.

The sulphate, for the sake of convenience, is referred to as one substance; actually, it is not. There are many unique, albeit structurally identical types of the compound — the most abundant in the body being chondroitin-4-sulphate and chondroitin-6-sulphate. The numbers for each are related to the location of the sulphate molecule, along the chondroitin sequence. It may be mentioned here that there is also a marginally different structure of chondroitin sulphate molecule — with each individual structure having different weights.

Researchers, however, don't have universal agreement on how different weights influence or promote absorption in the use of chondroitin compounds. Be that as it may, there is a general consensus that the lower the weight of the compound used, the more readily it is absorbed. This, of course, does not relate to what could be defined as "ideal" structure — one that could be thoroughly recommended for use.

First identified in the 1940s, as a component of cartilage, much of the early research with chondroitin was confined to animals — to observe, or evaluate, possible results of its application in joint health. As studies progressed, research on animals showed the ability of chondroitin in increasing proteoglycans production. This culminated in trials on human subjects. Results have been consistent: chondroitin relieves joint pain, improves mobility, reduces swelling in the affected part, and also one's "reliance" over NSAIDs.

Whatever the inference, the fact remains that chondroitin isn't as absorption-friendly in the body as glucosamine is. Less than ten per cent of chondroitin is absorbed vis-à-vis 90 per cent in the case of glucosamine. The issue is being debated and researched, and scientists are speculating how low-molecular mass chondroitin — available in the market — could be absorbed with better effect. While it is still scientific conjecture as to what happens after chondroitin is swallowed, studies, in general, have shown that the dietary supplement is more than equal to the task of providing better joint health and/or comfort.

THEY HELP REBUILD CARTILAGE

Glucosamine can help rebuild cartilage affected by osteoarthritis. When a capsule or tablet of the supplement is ingested, most of it ends up in the tissues of our joints. When glucosamine enters the chondrocytes — the cartilage-building assembly line inside the cartilage tissue — it is utilised to form new proteoglycans, which are responsible for healthy joint function. This by itself is a vital contribution, because in osteoarthritis the body's resources to manufacture adequate levels of new proteoglycans are depleted.

Ringing in the new, and ringing out the old, is nature's very own maxim in the cell-replacement process. This process is regulated and facilitated by enzymes that mortify the old cells. When this breakdown occurs more quickly, and replacement does not keep pace with it, just as quickly, the outcome is imminent — frail cartilage.

This situation calls for glucosamine intake. Glucosamine not only stalls the enzymatic destruction of proteoglycans, it also provides anti-inflammatory action to the affected joint.

MAGIC BULLET... OR?

Critics often say that glucosamine adherents have an ostentatious pitch: that the supplement has "the unique ability" to provide pain relief and help regenerate damaged tissue in joints. They ask: is this a marketing gimmick, or pitch — one you should run after and take?

Some even refer to glucosamine as nothing short of the "Gingko" of osteoarthritis therapy — a popular "natural" remedy. This is not without reason. In a survey of 2,146 primary care physicians and rheumatologists, and 90 patients, conducted by the respected *Arthritis Today* magazine, 34 per cent with the disease rated glucosamine as their favourite alternative to over-the-counter [OTC] pain medications. As a matter of fact, physicians/therapists rated its utility higher — with 45 per cent preferring to call glucosamine their "supplement" of choice.

However, not everyone is impressed by the beneficial effects of glucosamine. A section of rheumatologists [specialists in joint disorders] and researchers remains unconvinced, and adhere to one quip: that there have been no long-term clinical studies of the supplement in human beings. They also extend their cynicism to the fact that since glucosamine is a nutritional supplement, and, therefore, not regulated by the Food and Drug Administration [FDA], in the US — the regulation, of course, is not relevant, elsewhere — there can be no certainty, in quantifiable, measurable terms, regarding its potency or purity.

According to Timothy E McAlindon, an Assistant Professor of Medicine at The Arthritis Center, Boston University School of Medicine, US, and author of a topical study reviewing the scientific evidence about glucosamine and chondroitin, "The jury is still out on whether this works." Nevertheless, McAlindon and his colleagues agree that there is convincing evidence that "some glucosamine products" may actually help reduce inflammation and alleviate pain of osteoarthritis. But, what they are not clear about, at the moment, is whether glucosamine [and, chondroitin] can also "freeze" and "turn round" the disorder.

Other researchers maintain that a number of documented benefits may be exaggerated — or, that the conclusions of several studies were "inclined" and methodologically inconsistent. Some say, it is just the opposite. Their *raison d'être*: only one of the major 15 studies, researchers had, at one point of time, and thoroughly looked into, was sponsored by manufacturers and/or pharmaceutical companies.

However, in an article published in *Osteoarthritis and Cartilage*, principal investigator Amal K Das found that glucosamine/chondroitin sulphate dietary supplement [Cosamin DS] was effective in the management of joint pain in the knee. The randomised, placebo-controlled, peer-reviewed, clinical study was conducted on a 93-patient group, involving a combination of glucosamine and chondroitin sulphate and using a standardised index to measure joint pain. In the study, glucosamine/chondroitin supplements showed significant improvement in the management of joint pain in the knee. The response rate was 52 per cent in comparison to a 28 per cent response rate in the placebo group.

Briefly...

Glucosamine
• Increases the lubricating pattern in the joints
• Increases hydration of joints and tissues and, in so doing, reduces stiffness
• Stimulates the production of sugars that support the cartilage matrix
• Reduces the action of degradative enzymes that breakdown cartilage
• Activates anti-inflammatory characteristics.

Briefly...

Chondroitin
• Protects the health of joints, muscles, cartilage, ligaments and tendons
• Helps relieve inflamed joints associated with aging and osteoarthritis
• Promotes elasticity
• Shields the body against joint destruction
• Improves the body's natural ability to heal itself
• Acts as shock-absorber for the joints.

GLUCOSAMINE BETTER THAN OTHER TREATMENTS

Glucosamine sulphate versus NSAIDs [ibuprofen]

Clinical studies suggest that a definitive decrease in the intensity of osteoarthritis is almost a norm during the first week with the use of ibuprofen, but not with glucosamine sulphate. However, by the second week, as reported in most of the clinical trials, the glucosamine group holds on to its own — the result in terms of pain relief and osteoarthritic symptoms is apparent. Yet, the most important difference between NSAIDs and glucosamine is reflected by way of the former's side-effect profile.

In one study, one in three of the ibuprofen users complained of tummy upset; there were no reported side-effect symptoms from patients taking glucosamine sulphate. The supposition is relevant, although many of the studies were not extensive — the longest trial lasting two months. However, the overall pattern of results certainly shows promise in the use of glucosamine for the reduction of reported pain levels.

Oral Glucosamine sulphate versus placebo

In clinical trials, patients in the glucosamine sulphate group have often reported a significant decrease in pain and inflammation compared to the placebo group. Also, no adverse reactions were reported by patients, treated with glucosamine sulphate. This, experts opine, makes it an effective treatment option for osteoarthritis.

Glucosamine sulphate versus NSAIDs and placebo

In studies conducted in both NSAIDs and glucosamine sulphate groups of patients, each symptom of osteoarthritis improved, but to a much quicker and greater extent in the group treated with glucosamine. No placebo group has ever shown such results, or improvement.

Briefly...

Side-effects of NSAIDs
• Tummy ache, heartburn, and nausea
• Cartilage degeneration
• Leaky gut syndrome
• Cramps and diarrhoea
• Fluid retention and weight gain
• Drowsiness, dizziness, mental confusion
• Wounds bleed easily; they heal slowly
• Adverse reaction with alcohol
• Ringing in ears
• Lowered melatonin [a regulatory hormone] levels at night and body temperature.

Note: NSAIDs should be used with caution when taking certain herbs/herbal remedies.

Aspirin

Millions of people are taking the wonder drug, aspirin, on a daily basis. Aspirin has shown its efficacy to significantly reduce the risk of heart attack and stroke, and quell osteoarthritic pain. For some of its adherents, aspirin is a miracle remedy. But, one fact remains: for all its benefits, aspirin can also damage the lining of the gastro-intestinal tract. To alleviate the difficulty, a new, more-stomach-friendly aspirin called NCX-4016, which also encompasses the cyclooxygenase-2 [COX-2] inhibitor, celecoxib, is sold under the brand name, Celebrex, with promising results. The new aspirin, unlike its "old" model, releases nitric oxide, which increases blood flow into different parts of the body. Researchers feel that traditional aspirin probably causes damage to the stomach, because it may possibly reduce blood flow to the lining of the stomach. Experts reckon that nitric oxide, "triggered" by the new drug, which has run into rough weather due to its deleterious effects on patients with heart affections, opens up the blood flow, and may, therefore, protect the stomach lining.

Note: A new class of medications that were developed to manage the symptoms of arthritis without negative gastro-intestinal effects, COX-2 inhibitors stop the activity of specific cyclooxygenase [COX] enzymes, which release prostaglandins [responsible for pain and inflammation]. According to clinicians, the "old" NSAIDs inhibit both COX-2 — which causes inflammation — and, COX-1 — which promotes the healing of the gastric mucosa. COX-2 inhibitors, researchers reckon, inhibit only COX-2, not COX-1; they also affirm the gastric effects of the older NSAIDS. However, COX-2 drugs come with a host of other problems; as a matter of fact, *The Journal of the American Medical Association* has released a special communiqué warning patients that the new COX-2 inhibitors increased the occurrence of heart attack, stroke and blood clots, in certain patients.

****

Chapter 5

HOW GLUCOSAMINE WORKS

Things are a-changin' for glucosamine; it is no longer a question why one has not heard about it yet. The fact is many progressive doctors/therapists today are prescribing glucosamine sulphate for osteoarthritis. But, the problem, or ticklish question, we encounter is the label — glucosamine is classified as a nutritional supplement, not a drug. Hence, it may be an out-of-pocket expenditure, in some countries — not in the UK, for example, where it is available on NHS [National Health Service].

In addition to subjective clinical studies, which detractors point out as not being substantial, or all-embracing, it may also be mentioned that most studies offer data on the basis of animal-based clinical trials performed to evaluate how glucosamine works. It has, however, been found that *in vitro* [test tubes outside the body, and not inside the body], glucosamine sulphate stimulates cartilage cells to synthesise glycosaminoglycans and proteoglycans.

Oral glucosamine sulphate has had beneficial effects on inflammation and joint pain, in animal studies. However, one question still remains: how do glucosamine supplements, taken orally, really get to the right place in the joint to stimulate new cartilage growth, as many pro-glucosamine bodies maintain.

In an article published in *The Journal of the American Medical Association* [JAMA], a group of participants was given glucosamine sulphate tagged with a radioactive dye. The objective was simple. The technique allowed investigators to follow the glucosamine "trail" through the body. The results showed that oral glucosamine sulphate became a component of cartilage, supporting all of the subjective results experienced and reported by patients, from time to time.

GROWING DISENCHANTMENT WITH CONVENTIONAL TREATMENT

Although the two supplements have been in vogue as a means of primary treatment in Europe, they have made their presence felt in the US, and elsewhere, recently, and with good effect. The reason for this development is not difficult to understand.

Pharmaceutical companies often spend their resources, not just in terms of money, or inclination, researching and marketing drugs — like NSAIDs — to treat diseases. This is also where their organised "action" bears fruit — getting patents for their drugs. Besides this, patented medicines help them recover their enormous investments. Furthermore, it helps them protect, garner, even conquer, markets and/or charge prices higher than those manufactured by their competitors.

Not that the drive for patents is "bad" medicine. It is good, because it gives the lead to the development of more useful and life-saving medications. But, there is a downside to the idea — nutritional supplements, like glucosamine and chondroitin, cannot be patented. Hence, pharmaceutical companies have little interest in them. This also explains why most companies in the pharmaceutical business hanker for new [patented] drugs that bring in wealth, even if they cause adverse side-effects in patients using them.

The incongruity is perceptible. Funding is a difficult word for research efforts for nutritional supplements — even if they sound as glamorous as patented medicines by their names. Though this does not in any way detract from the merits of their amazing, sometimes miraculous healing properties, nutritional supplements don't really attract a first-rate budget for their development — one that would put drug research to shame. Also, the whopping investment on "adverteasements," if not advertisements, is another "knob" that gives top pharmaceutical companies the cutting-edge not to speak of its reach to tap prospective customers, which supplements cannot match.

On the upside, things are now changing — not because enthusiasm has grown for natural supplements, and this has led to money coming in for research. Far from it. Thanks to the ubiquitous nature and reach of the Internet, and disenchantment with conventional medicine, there seems to be a growing hunger for information on natural supplements, especially glucosamine and chondroitin, among patients, and the public at large — besides conventional and alternative physicians.

MORE ON CHONDROITIN

Chondroitin is quite akin to glucosamine in its beneficial function. It also plays a similar, or complementary, role. Besides, it ushers in a new era of "crop" production — in this case, healthy, water-trapping proteoglycans.

Chondroitin has a negative charge. This explains why each of its molecules is drawn away from nearby molecules to make room for water to fill within the cartilage structure. While laboratory studies suggest that both the supplements "boost" the creation of proteoglycans, the absorption of water into the cartilage is just as important a factor. Cartilage, as you may, perhaps, know has no blood supply of its own; it has to, therefore, depend to a large extent on the movement of fluids to direct necessary nutrients into the joint. This is what we called the "shock-absorber effect," caused during joint movement, earlier in this book.

You will also recall that certain enzymes destroy proteoglycans to "loop" in new ones. In osteoarthritis, these enzymes are "out of bounds" with new proteoglycans. It is precisely here that chondroitin plays a significant role. Chondroitin stalls and slows down the imbalance caused by the death of proteoglycans and collagen in cartilage.

A study in Italy, to cull just one example, showed the use of oral chondroitin sulphate for a period of five days by a group of individuals, with cartilage degeneration, and another with healthy cartilage, to significantly decrease the levels of degradation in both groups.

Chondroitin, like glucosamine, has the wherewithal to decrease joint inflammation — which reaches alarming levels as the osteoarthritic disease progresses and debilitates the affected individual. The best part is: the two supplements do not alter or harm prostaglandins, the hormone-like substances or natural chemicals, which are involved in inflammation, unlike NSAIDs, which alter them and also cause side-effects, such as tummy distress.

CHONDROITIN AND RISK OF MAD COW DISEASE? NO WAY!

There are quite a few techniques used for the extraction of chondroitin sulphate. The transformation of cow trache into cartilage powder was one detailed method. The process used was hammer milling, followed by acid-pepsin digestion to remove the bovine [cow] protein, along with acetone extraction to eliminate the fat. The pure cartilage was, thereafter, pulverised by ball milling into micro-particles that averaged about 60 micron in size. This fine powder was dried on large racks and tested for chemical content and bacteriological purity. Too extensive a process, isn't it? Besides, experts feared that this practice, in spite of safeguards in place, was not without risks — because, it was "theoretically" possible for bovine spongiform encephalopathy [BSE], a serious disease affecting cows, to be transmitted through cow-derived products — to strike humans in its alternative form, variant Creutzfeldt-Jakob Disease [vCJD].

Not any more. So, forget about the danger.

Today, you have chondroitin sulphate products made from shark cartilage; besides, companies are moving towards making sure they use the ingredient for all chondroitin products in the future. So, relax — and, don't hold your breath. Because, chondroitin sulphate, made from shark cartilage is not only safe, but also trustworthy.

REMODELLING THE JOINTS

The two supplements, glucosamine and chondroitin, restore the joint modelling process and elevate balance — balance holds the key to stopping osteoarthritis from running wild. Besides, they prop up the proteoglycans' building, or re-building, ability, aside from chondrocytes. In a major [double-blind] study, reported in *The Lancet*, the respected British medical journal, researchers from four countries found convincing evidence that glucosamine had the ability to prevent osteoarthritic progression in 212 subjects. A double-blind study is a clinical trial in which neither the study staff nor the participants know which participants are receiving the experimental substance, and who are receiving a placebo, or another therapy. Double-blind trials are thought to produce objective results, since the researchers' and volunteers' expectations about the experimental substance do not affect the outcome.

The study was no quick "mug-shot" at glucosamine; it was based on sound scientific principles and adhered to the strictest norms. That's not all. Neither the patients nor medical professionals had a ghost of an idea, or clue, as to who among the trial group was taking glucosamine and/or placebo. The study was also without bias, because there is always the prospect of detracting from the merits of any benefit as having emerged due to "straight-line" thinking, or wishful contemplation.

The patients in the study were all afflicted with osteoarthritis of the knee joint. Exactly half of the individuals took 1,500 mg of glucosamine sulphate per day; the other half was given placebo. The supplement "diet" went on for a period of three years, and the end-result was encouraging. Pain dropped by 20-25 per cent among the subjects taking glucosamine; symptoms increased by 10 per cent in the placebo group. X-ray studies also substantiated the progress — the glucosamine group showed no deterioration in their knee-joint abnormalities, whereas the placebo group continued to experience worsening abnormalities. This was a groundbreaking outcome, even though it did not necessarily excite researchers who had already concurred that glucosamine was able to help the cartilage rebuild itself — with the aid of scanned electron micrographs. The experience was quite similar with patients taking chondroitin supplements. When an adult group of 226, with thinning cartilage, was given oral doses of chondroitin and placebo, for a period of one year, the cartilage in the former not only stopped thinning, but also improved its thickness. Besides this, the group also showed adequate improvement in pain and joint mobility, including other parameters.

In a review published in JAMA, which was based on [re]analysis of research conducted over a three-decade period [1966-1999], researchers concluded that the two supplements do, in fact, show[ed] a "moderate-to-large" effect for alleviating symptoms of osteoarthritis...

The two reports, emerge as they do from two prestigious journals, are not just suggestive, but also indicative, of the fact that glucosamine and chondroitin are resolute, and fairly safe, contenders in the long-term management of osteoarthritis.

The real shot in the arm for the two supplements emerged, thanks to the reception they received from Drs Jason Theodosakis, Brian Adderly, and Barry Fox's landmark 1997 book, *The Arthritis Cure*. The book contended, in clear terms, the medical fact that glucosamine and chondroitin could halt, reverse, and even offer a cure for osteoarthritis. Soon enough, the two supplements became as big a name as the newest, or latest, blockbuster movie from Hollywood and/or Bollywood.

It is, of course, quite easy for one to go overboard in view of the fact that the two supplements seem to break new ground with every realistic trial. It would also be no exaggeration to say that many highly qualified and respected researchers have gone on record, despite their usual scientific inclination for discretion, and recommend that it would be useful to try the two-supplement-option prior to the use of aspirin, NSAIDs, or surgery.

Researchers, however, assert that this is no fail-safe start; they also caution that this is no total solution to taking the osteoarthritic bull by its horns. However, what they espouse is that glucosamine and chondroitin are the most sensible options to begin with — and, for two reasons. Their potential to provide ample benefit to the patient is high; at the same time, the two also have relatively minimal side-effect profile. In other words, they are safe.

SAFETY AND BETTER MOBILITY

For those used to taking ibuprofen, the NSAID pain reliever, and experiencing relief within a week's time, a short course on glucosamine/chondroitin isn't going to give quick results or benefit.

The two supplements are slow starters, but when they get into you, after one full month of use, the results are often dramatic. It is rightly said that what takes time to heal heals best. The two supplements work at a level that NSAIDs don't; they go to the root cause of the osteoarthritic problem, rebuild the joint structure, and provide the platform to create new, healthy tissue — a process that has to be time-consuming.

In a 2003 study, conducted by lead researcher, Florent Richy, an epidemiologist with the University of Liege, Belgium, researchers analysed data from 15 studies of glucosamine/chondroitin compounds. They found that these "nutrients" do work on symptoms — and provide mobility, pain relief, and better quality of life — and, that they are very safe.

The studies in Richy's analysis all focused on osteoarthritis of the knee, and on studies of 1,775 patients — 1,020 taking glucosamine and 755 taking chondroitin — which showed "significant changes" in the symptoms of patients taking them. No placebo group showed this kind of improvement.

Richy's findings suggested that glucosamine significantly improved joint space narrowing. In addition, two chondroitin studies showed comparable results, and indicated that both supplements significantly reduced symptoms such as pain, stiffness, physical functioning, and joint mobility. Symptom improvement began about two weeks after starting the supplements.
 Research also suggests that taking at least 1,500 mg/day of oral glucosamine sulphate for three years was most effective in slowing the degenerative process. As regards chondroitin, the findings are, more or less, similar, if not as clear-cut. However, according to Richy, the overall safety of glucosamine and chondroitin can be considered excellent. There are, he contends, substantial beneficial

effects on symptoms of glucosamine and chondroitin therapy when compared with placebo.

The two supplements also reduce the swelling of the inflamed joint and morning stiffness — or, when the joint has been inactive for a while. Those who take glucosamine/chondroitin indicate that they are able to move their affected joint better; many have also reported improved walking activity.

These are some of the obvious benefits of taking the two supplements, though the decision to take or not to take them is individual, or personal, choice. However, one fact remains: osteoarthritis, if not treated, is a progressive degenerative condition, which only gets worse as time rolls by. The idea of not doing anything at all holds enormous risk.

All the same, the use of glucosamine/chondroitin therapy in osteoarthritis is aimed at decreasing pain and helping to maintain or improve joint function. While the pharmacological treatment of osteoarthritis has included the use of aspirin, acetaminophen, and NSAIDs, studies in the recent past have investigated, and deduced, the potential role of chondroprotective [cartilage-protecting] agents, like the two supplements, in repairing articular cartilage and slowing down the degenerative process of osteoarthritis.

Glucosamine has gained extensive popularity in the treatment of osteoarthritic conditions, including usage in preventative treatment. Though some experts are incredulous of its value vis-à-vis OTC supplements, many patients and newly validated, but not substantially diverse, studies have turned the tide — even if they are not sizeable — in the supplement's favour, by reporting excellent symptomatic relief, comparable to any NSAID drug. And, again, without NSAIDs' side-effects portrait.

Chapter 6

GETTING IT RIGHT...

Treatment of osteoarthritis is two-fold: symptom-modifying and structure-modifying. Regrettably, no conventional medical prescription, or OTC medication, has been found to be effective in the latter. The standard use of NSAIDs is nothing but palliative — just a step short of masquerading some of the symptoms of osteoarthritis. What's more, some of the NSAIDs now in use are actually known to worsen, not modify, the course of the disease.

NSAIDs give pain relief by blocking the production of prostaglandins. Prostaglandins are hormone-like substances that can prompt inflammation. However, by "jamming" prostaglandins, NSAIDs do more harm than good. This is, in other words, the basis of their side-effects. Besides this, NSAIDs have also been shown to cause ulcers, because they hinder the function of prostaglandins, which control the secretion of gastric juices and the mucous layer that lines the stomach. Worse still, NSAIDs also cause gastro-intestinal bleeding and kidney failure. Reports indicate that NSAIDs-induced haemorrhages in the US alone, for instance, have lead to over 125,000 hospitalisations, including hundreds of deaths.

Long-term use of NSAIDs has also been reported to accelerate cartilage destruction. In other words, they seem to cause great harm than "treating" osteoarthritis. They suppress the disease, and do not go deep into the root of the problem. This isn't an option that you'd be happy to bargain for. Right?

... AND PERFECT

It is in situations such as those outlined above that glucosamine and chondroitin score yet another triumph. The two supplements not only have the ability to "swing" a coup of sorts: they also play their role as symptom-modifying and structure-modifying agents with profound effect. They ease the symptoms of osteoarthritis, yes; they also transform the structural composites of the joint.

Just the right thing to do to stifle bone discomfort and mend the joint? Indeed.

In a nutshell, glucosamine and chondroitin offer their users the following discernable benefits:

- Ease joint pain and swelling
- Enhance the water content of cartilage
- Slow down the power of cartilage-swallowing enzymes
- Establish the production of new proteoglycans and collagen components
- Augment viscosity of the synovial fluid for joint lubrication.

BETTER FOR SURE

Studies have also suggested that glucosamine is as effective as ibuprofen for symptomatic relief of osteoarthritis. A group of 200 participants with osteoarthritis of the knee joint took part in a one-month study. Half of the group took 1,500 mg of glucosamine daily; the other 100 took 1,200 mg of ibuprofen.

The investigators recorded symptoms such as pain at night, pain after immobility, after standing, and after rising from chair, including walking distance and limitation of day-to-day activities, as a single score on the Lequesne Index — a research tool used to measure the severity of osteoarthritic symptoms. The study found glucosamine to be as effective as conventional drug therapy, but without the harmful side-effects of NSAIDs.

HALTING CARTILAGE DESTRUCTION

Glucosamine, a natural sugar, which is bound to protein [Diabetics — there is no need to push the panic-button!] — is made from chitin, derived from shellfish, or shark cartilage. A key component of the extracellular matrix of cartilage, glucosamine has charged side chains, which absorb water and provide lubrication and shock-absorption for the cartilage that covers the ends of the bones in the joints.

In osteoarthritis, glucosamine and other "sugars" decline in concentration and lose some of their ability to absorb water. Taking glucosamine supplements has, therefore, shown to improve cartilage function and offer relief from pain as effectively as ibuprofen in double-blind prospective trials.

Conventional treatment for osteoarthritis affects the symptoms, but not the disease. Glucosamine has been investigated as a possible disease-modifying supplement because, after ingestion, it has been shown to get absorbed in the joints. In addition, since it is a key component of the extracellular framework of cartilage, there are some prospective double-blind studies showing its equivalence to non-steroidal anti-inflammatory drugs [NSAIDs].

Glucosamine could have well been the first effective, or basic, therapy for osteoarthritis. When researchers began to seriously probe the substance for its healing properties, in the mid-1960s, the work did not turn out to be as exciting as the emerging healing effects and positive results. As research progressed, even if it was "sloppy," to critics, the conventional school of medicine largely ignored claims, and thought of controlled clinical trials of glucosamine — which led to uniform findings that it relieves pain as effectively as NSAIDs — as a waste of time.

This despite the fact that glucosamine [sulphate] naturally occurs in our body, and is almost free of toxic effects. However, there is now some support in sections of the medical community that the substance has perceptible chondroprotective properties and is suitable for long-term therapeutic use. This relative "backing" has not deterred researchers — who see more than a glimmer of scientific hope in the healing properties of the substance — in their quest to establish glucosamine supplement treatment as a strong, acceptable line of healing.

The end is far from over, and it is not possible to predict who will win the "race." But, a long scientific journey into the realms of finding out an appropriate statement to address the issue was a mixed bag. The essential of the essentials in the glucosamine/chondroitin fulcrum was put to the litmus, if not ultimate, test in a $14-million study — The Glucosamine/Chondroitin Arthritis Intervention Trial [GAIT] — set up by the National Center for Complementary and Alternative Medicine and the National Institute of Arthritis and Musculoskeletal Disease, US.

The study examined whether glucosamine and chondroitin do, indeed, relieve the pain of osteoarthritis. The study enrolled over 1,600 patients, for twenty-four weeks, in as many as thirteen different clinical centres. This was followed by a subset of participating subjects for another eighteen months. Needless to say, the study measured, in actual terms, the efficacy of the two supplements, separately and in combination, and compared results with celecoxib [a conventional COX-2 medicine] for alleviating osteoarthritic knee pain.

The study results implied that the two supplements could possibly work in mild-to-moderate osteoarthritis — and, also, perhaps, just marginally improve your quality of life. You be the judge.

58

THE REVOLUTION

In the early part of the book, we had looked at the causes of primary osteoarthritis — such as aging, genetic factors, malnutrition, free radicals stress, and constant or repetitive strain on joints. However, it must be mentioned that age alone does not cause the disorder. It is established that the chemical composition of cartilage in osteoarthritic patients resembles the pattern seen in children.

There is, of course, considerable evidence that the combined effects of the factors cited hamper the body's ability to renew the key chemical components of cartilage. The most critical loss being the body's inability to make adequate amounts of glycosaminoglycans — especially glucosamine sulphate — an essential structural constituent of cartilage tissues. This suggests why the substance could be actively considered as the first therapeutic agent capable of halting cartilage destruction in osteoarthritis.

To maintain the natural resiliency of cartilage, our body must be able to replenish and smarten up chondroitin sulphate molecules and proteoglycans. Otherwise, the rate of decay, especially in primary osteoarthritis, will exceed the tempo of repair.

It is exactly here that glucosamine and chondroitin score yet another victory for you.

DEPENDABLE OPTION

It may be a common practice for one to ascertain the quality of the drug you are required to take — you'd find out with your doctor, especially if you are not familiar with the standing, or reputation, of the company that has manufactured it. Else, it does not worry you. This may not be possible with supplements — in their capsule/tablet form, or any other presentation.

You may ask yourself: "How am I to know its genuine nature, or quality?" Rest assured — there isn't anything to lose your sleep on. Most of the companies that manufacture supplements, like glucosamine and chondroitin, have a clean bill of health — though it has been a common practice for them to blame each other for marketing "poor-quality" products.

In a survey conducted in the US, over twenty-five brands of glucosamine were put to the test. The medicinal bottles were purchased, at random, from health stores, and sent to independent laboratories for analysis. The result was assuring — every single product/bottle contained exactly what the label purported its buyer to believe.

COST BENEFITS

Pharmaceutical companies spend a whopping US$15-billion for arthritis research and medicines annually — and, the results, to this day, have not really totally "cured" ailing joints, as much as sales figures for drugs sold. On the other hand, figures indicate that people who are on the two-supplement diet spend around a good US$600 million — which actually pales in comparison vis-à-vis the latter. What's more important is costs of glucosamine and chondroitin are coming down, thanks to competition in the marketplace.

This is not all. A typical monthly regimen on a branded NSAID could cost you approximately £60 [US$110]; if it is generic, the costs may be about £24 [US$45]. Compare it with what you would spend for the two supplements — a 30-day supply of a combination product [1,500 mg of glucosamine sulphate, and 1,200 mg of chondroitin sulphate] may reduce your bill by £20 [US$40]. This isn't a bargain, or compromise. The brands available in the market have been tested, as already cited, and hold a reputation that is second to none.

The final score is apparent: glucosamine and chondroitin offer you not just economy, or affordable costs, but they also help your sore joint and you won't feel the pinch of an expensive monthly bill.

Call it a "joint-healing" process that is light on the wallet and also safe.

****

Chapter 7

HOW TO ACHIEVE MAXIMUM RELIEF

The preceding chapters would have given you enough food for thought for trying the two supplements with the objective of giving your joints obvious benefits. However, what may bother you to an extent or degree is how you could derive maximum relief. In other words, make sure that you are taking the right form of the two supplements that suits your specific needs. There is no reason to worry — the following summary provides the information that you are looking for.

Glucosamine is available in three forms: the sulphate form, which you have already read about, glucosamine hydrochloride [HCl], and N-acetyl glucosamine. Though the sulphate form has been extensively studied, the other two forms have also been analysed and results of their positive attributes in effective treatment have emerged. What is, however, lacking is scientific data comparing them — if one of them is better than the other. If ever there was a supplement of choice from the glucosamine family, the sulphate form would get the thumbs-up sign — because, it has been the most researched and quantified. Also, there is a school of thought that recommends a combination of the three products — so that you derive the best of all the "three worlds."

As far as chondroitin is concerned, there isn't anything as complex. The supplement is generally available in the sulphate form. Also, studies have established the efficacy of low-weight chondroitin, because the lower-weight compounds are more easily absorbed. It is agreed that the compounds differ marginally in terms of where the sulphate element is attached to the chondroitin molecule — as has been explained elsewhere in the book. All you need to do is, of course, look at the label carefully, and make sure you buy the best product available.

Absorption of chondroitin appears to occur from the stomach and small intestine.

SULPHUR "SPRING"

It would only be prudent for us to find out the reason why the sulphate form in either supplement offers the best form of treatment. Sulphate is a form of sulphur — an essential nutrient needed for the stabilisation of the connective tissue matrix as well as the manufacture of collagen. When sulphate levels of the body are low, or drop down, the manufacture of the complex compounds, glycosaminoglycans — the polysaccharides in proteoglycans — is interfered with. This is a major setback in patients with osteoarthritis. Joints affected by osteoarthritis have an increased need for glycosaminoglycans — and, when the need is not fulfilled, there may not be enough sulphate available to manufacture them. Get the point? Add glucosamine and chondroitin sulphate to your daily "to-take" list, and your sulphate requirement would be taken care of, with good effect.

G&C COMPARED

It may be understandable why some researchers believe that it would make sense for one to take both glucosamine and chondroitin sulphate in combination form, because they perform complementary functions in the cartilage. Interestingly, a few clinical trials have demonstrated superior results by the use of glucosamine alone; besides this, the supplement is inexpensive.

Though agreement is divided on whether or not chondroitin can add value to glucosamine treatment, it is quite clear that the former plays a definitive role in critical metabolic functions having therapeutic uses. It attracts, like glucosamine, water into the cartilage matrix to stimulate the production of glycosaminoglycans, proteoglycans, and collagen. What also makes it stand out is its ability to prevent enzymes from dissolving the cartilage and depriving it of nutrients — a function which isn't glucosamine's forte.

There is, however, a feeling in the medical community that our body does not need supplemental chondroitin as much as glucosamine, since it is made up of linked glucosamine sulphate molecules. Also, glucosamine alone is enough to stimulate the synthesis of chondroitin by chondrocytes. Some researchers also suggest that chondroitin has not been subject to a "heavy" battery of clinical trials yet — and, that most of its verifiable results have been achieved with injections of the molecule [or, in laboratory animals]. The consensus today is: it would be sensible for one to take glucosamine for a period of two months, and elicit if discernable benefits are achieved — before taking supplemental chondroitin sulphate.

All the same, there is emerging opinion on the valuable benefits of taking a combination product. Some researchers have found that the two, in unison, provide a "synergistic" effect and benefit to the joint — an outcome that exceeds the benefits provided by one supplement at a time. Their reasoning is simple: glucosamine stimulates the production of glycosaminoglycans, while chondroitin impedes their breakdown. The outcome: a greater quantity of healthy cartilage.

In addition, supplements of glucosamine HCl and low-weight chondroitin sulphate, and vitamin-mineral complexes [e.g., manganese ascorbate], have been tested singly, and in combination, to show how well each of these nutritional supplements slowed down the process of cartilage degeneration in rabbits.

WHO SHOULD TAKE

Individuals who have been diagnosed with osteoarthritis by a doctor should consider taking glucosamine and chondroitin. It does not matter whether your treatment regimen with NSAIDs has given you relief from pain. The reason is simple: you'd take the two supplements to prevent an aggravation of the disease at a later date. Also, there is no reason for you to wait for an event of this nature to happen, and then call your two-supplement ammo into action.

It is not that if one has no apparent sign or symptom of osteoarthritis s/he should refrain from taking them. People after the age of 65 are suitable candidates — because, they have a three per cent greater risk of developing the disease on a yearly basis. Younger people who are at risk should also take it — especially, if they play any sport, perform repetitive activities, or are overweight/obese.

It is not that this "forewarned-is-forearmed" prophylactic therapy is going to offer you an insurance policy, but it is better to be wise before the event, not after — more so, if you have any of the known risk factors for osteoarthritis, viz., previous joint injuries, genetic or family predisposition, and obesity.

Who should not...
- Glucosamine, or chondroitin, should not be taken, if you are pregnant, or could become pregnant
- Glucosamine, or chondroitin, should not be taken if you are breast-feeding. Also, children should not take glucosamine or chondroitin.

EASE OF USE

Glucosamine and chondroitin sulphate supplements are available in pharmacies, health food stores etc., without a prescription, in capsule/tablet form. Hence, they are easy to carry and take.

Gone are the days when you had to carry a bottle of glucosamine 500 mg capsules/tablets/pills, and pop them up wherever you were, three times, during the course of the day. New research has shown that taking a 1,500 mg pill, once a day, is as effective as divided doses; may be, better. Also, the idea is convenient: no need to stock the pill in your carry bag, or briefcase. This also holds good for chondroitin sulphate 800 mg, once-a-day pill, instead of the 400 mg twice-daily pill.

Most important — the supplements are well accepted by the body, and they are safe.

****

Chapter 8

VITAMINS, MINERALS AND OTHER SUPPLEMENTS

It is quite well known that osteoarthritis patients are deficient in key nutrients, vitamins and minerals. Though it is not clear whether deficiencies contribute to OA, or there are extra-nutritional demands imposed by chronic inflammation, it makes sense for osteoarthritis patients to take an adequate intake of select nutrients.

The most useful nutrients are vitamins C, D, and E, aside from boron, selenium, and zinc. May be, you could try a multivitamin supplement that offers all the nutrients — with their appropriate doses provided and taken care of. However, it would be wise to exercise caution while taking these pills, because excess dosage may increase other health risks. For instance, high vitamin A intake could harm auto-immune activity, just as much as excess daily doses [>100 milligram] of zinc may lead to detrimental changes in blood cholesterol. [RDA = Recommended Daily Allowance]

Vitamin	RDA*	Function	Food Sources	Safe Supplement Level
Vitamin A	800 RE	Growth, vision, anti-oxidant, healthy mucous membrane	Organ meats, milk, oysters, mackerel	Can be toxic, do not exceed safe level: 1,000 RE
Beta-carotene	10-30 mg**	Boosts immunity, anti-oxidant, precursor to vitamin A	Dark orange, bright green, red fruits and vegetables	Non-toxic form of vitamin A: 30-50 mg

Vitamin	RDA*	Function	Food Sources	Safe Supplement Level
Vitamin D	200 IU	Helps build bones and teeth, maintains muscles and nerves, prevents skin disorders	Sunlight, fish with small bones, fortified milk, shrimp	Toxic, if taken in doses of more than 4 x RDA: **400 IU**
Vitamin E	12 IU or 8 mg	Slows down aging; anti-oxidant; helps in preventing cancer and heart disease. Helps in decreasing symptoms of lupus, a joint affection.	Safflower oil, wheat germ, peaches, spinach	Non-toxic: **200-400 mg**
Vitamin B6	1.6 mg	Metabolism of carbohydrates, fat, and protein. Required for the manufacturing of hormones and haemoglobin. Functioning of central nervous system.	Banana, avocado, beef, chicken, fish, leafy greens.	Toxic [though this is debatable] to nervous system, if greater than 200 mg: **10 mg**
Folic Acid	180-400 mcg	Helps regulate cell division and transfer Production of neuro-transmitters.	Brewers' yeast, liver, legumes, orange juice, and dark leafy greens.	Non-toxic: **400 mcg**

Vitamin	RDA*	Function	Food Sources	Safe Supplement Level
Vitamin C	**60 mg**	Forms collagen, promotes healing, and acts as an anti-oxidant.	Citrus fruits and juices. Strawberries, cantaloupe, tomato juice, potato, and broccoli.	Non-toxic: **1,000-2,000 mg**

- RDA based on adults.
- ** No RDA has been established [Recommendation made by the Alliance on Aging].

Adapted, from and, by courtesy of: Kay G Mullin, RD, Sports Nutritionist, Stone Clinic.

Note: There are reports that suggest that some glucosamine supplements contain the mineral, manganese, in excess. Although studies confirm no report of manganese toxicity [cough, high blood pressure, anaemia, nervous disorders, tremor and weakness], it is better to exercise caution while buying the product.

Other supplements that can be taken with glucosamine include niacinamide [vitamin B3], which is said to be particularly effective in relieving knee pain; the ancient ayurvedic remedy, boswellia, a gummy tree resin, is another, that has a proven clinical record to inhibit inflammation and help build cartilage.

Sea cucumber has been attributed to have healing properties in osteoarthritis. Some recommend the use of Chinese herbal remedies that may, through unknown mechanisms, reduce pain and stiffness and boost grip strength.

One form of the amino acid methionine, SAMe [S-adenosylmethionine] has anti-inflammatory effects similar to ibuprofen, and has been shown to rebuild cartilage. Gelatin [containing the amino acids, glycine and proline], emu oil, and other joint-building nutrients, may also be worth trying, if other measures fail; however, far too little is known about their actual effectiveness.

All the same, any of these remedies may be used along with topically applied cayenne cream for pain relief. The capsaicin — the hot chemical in chillies — in cayenne inhibits production of substance P, a chemical involved in sending pain messages to the brain. Initial applications, however, may cause a burning sensation.

Turmeric, the good, old traditional Indian remedy, has also been found to be useful. The reason being curcumin, the main active ingredient in turmeric, has anti-inflammatory properties. Another ancient and useful remedy is ginger, with its known anti-inflammatory properties.

Fish oils

Fish oils, including their chemical cousins found in plants [flaxseed], are among the greatest nutritional chronicles of our time. The oils in specific plants and fish are so important that they are called essential fatty acids [EFAs]. Specific fatty acids modify inflammation and help treat conditions such as osteoarthritis. Besides being critical for the development of nerve and brain function in infants, fish oils are absorbed directly into the outer fatty layer of every cell, where they act like "cellular cushion," or wall, protecting each cell from the outside environment. Fats, in recent history, have become a distasteful expression. However, in actuality, fats are life's lubricants and powerhouses of energy. The human body need fats for optimal health. This is not all: women, in particular, need fats to build their hormones. May be, the correct turn of phrase would be: we need fats, yes; but, we need to keep a tab on their intake.

FREE RADICALS: KNOCKIN' THEM OUT

Anti-oxidants are of utmost importance for anyone with osteoarthritis. As you may already know, any inflammatory process releases a large number of harmful compounds called free radicals. A free radical, in such a situation, is depleted of one of its electrons, a very vital part. In a move to restore balance, the free radical reacts with any molecule, including the DNA, in its immediate vicinity. The result is a dangerous game — as the original free radical "pilfers" an electron from another molecule, it causes that particular molecule to become unstable. This leads to a chain reaction — however, the need to establish stability does not really happen. Anti-oxidants act as the umpire in the body, and can stall this potentially dangerous distraction. This explains why when free radicals are left uncontrolled, they can just as well devastate the body.

Vitamin E is a very important anti-oxidant in our body's defence mechanism in its war against free radicals. As one study reports, patients with osteoarthritis took 600 mg of vitamin E on a daily basis, or a placebo for 10 days; and, vice versa. Half of the patients on vitamin E reported reduced pain, as against four per cent in the placebo group. Studies have also compared the efficacy of vitamin E with diclofenac, a NSAID. Results indicate that the former seems to be as effective as the latter for improving joint mobility and "walk-time."

Vitamin C is another great anti-oxidant that has been found to offer observable relief in osteoarthritis. Studies have shown that it can provide a three-fold less risk in the progression of the disease, and in its various stages. Some researchers relate to the utility value of vitamin C, a water-soluble vitamin, better than fat-soluble vitamins like vitamin E or beta-carotene. The implication is clear: the watery environment of certain parts of the joint is inclined to benefit more from a water-soluble vitamin.

Some authorities also recommend the use of bioflavonoids, such as quercetin and proanthocyanidins, found in pine bark and grape seed extract, as also being useful in preventing accumulation of fluids, swelling, and joint pains.

MSM AND SAMe: NEW AIDS

MSM [methylsulphonylmethane], a natural form of organic sulphur, is found in all living organisms, including human body fluids and tissues. Robert Herschler and Stanley Jacob of the University of Oregon Medical School, US, isolated it, in the early 1980s. The duo's research showed that MSM is a natural sulphur compound, and also one of the most important compounds in our bodies, and just as vital as water and sodium. Further studies also demonstrated that the sulphur present in MSM, called sulphonyl, was safe, and as essential as vitamin C in our diet. However this may be, MSM, a member of the sulphur family, should not be confused with sulpha drugs, which some people are allergic to.

A fragrance-free, water-soluble, white crystalline material that supplies a bioavailable form of dietary sulphur, MSM originates in the ocean and reaches the human food chain through rainfall. MSM is also found in many common foods, including raw milk, meat, fish, and a variety of fruits, vegetables, and grains. However, it is normally lost from our food by heating, storage, processing, drying, cooking, preserving, and even washing. While the substance has been shown to add elasticity to cell walls by allowing fluids to pass through the tissue more easily, it has also been found that it can increase tissue pliability and promote the repair of damaged skin.

74

Our MSM levels reduce with age; this results in symptoms of fatigue, tissue and organ malfunction, and increased susceptibility to disease. In one preliminary study, ten osteoarthritis patients taking MSM were compared with six who took a placebo. Results indicated almost 80 per cent control of pain within the first six weeks in them, while only two patients showed minimal improvement [less than 20 per cent] on placebo.

MSM has also been favoured to be a natural remedy for osteoarthritis, tendonitis and bursitis, muscular soreness and athletic injuries, carpal tunnel syndrome [which is caused by the compression of the median nerve in the wrist — usually the result of repetitive motion of the wrist; e.g., computer use], post-traumatic inflammation and pain, heartburn and hyperacidity, headaches and back pain, and allergies. Researchers say that those taking MSM may notice other benefits — softer skin, harder nails, thicker hair, and softening of scar tissue. An allotted time of about a month, they add, may be needed before significant improvement is seen, with the use of MSM.

MSM, researchers point out, is safe. In a survey conducted at the Oregon Health Sciences University, US, patients who received oral MSM, as part of their treatment, showed no toxic build-up, even after years of taking more than 2,000 mg of MSM each day. Experts recommend patients to take MSM in pill or liquid form, though the substance is also available in topical formulas. It may be remarked that MSM topical creams may not be worth trying, because the heating process may destroy the bioavailability of MSM. A body of opinion also favours the use of MSM with other natural compounds, because MSM has the ability to allow fluids to pass through the tissue more easily. This can lead to better absorption.

The use of glucosamine and MSM for the use of symptom reduction and tissue repair in joints is preferred in some of the scientific literature today, thanks mainly due to their low percentage of side-effects [Side-effects, even if they occur, are often mild in nature and controllable].

Topical formulas are also thought of as a good option by some prescribers. When they are combined with a good delivery system, they offer local transfer of ingredients directly to the site of annoyance. However, it will be some time before studies, which are now in progress, can offer us a better understanding of the process and also better treatment plans.

SAMe [S-adenosylmethionine], like MSM, is also a natural product that has been proven to offer many benefits in osteoarthritis. In addition, it appears to promote production of cartilage proteoglycans, and is, therefore, therapeutically beneficial in osteoarthritis in well-controlled oral doses. Needless to say, SAMe and other safe nutritional measures, which support proteoglycans synthesis, may offer a practical means of preventing or delaying the onset of osteoarthritis in older people or athletes.

One of the most preferred supplements in the market, SAMe is not an herb, hormone, vitamin, or "nutrient" *per se*. In the human body, SAMe is also known to be essential for maintaining the structure of cell membranes and manufacturing substances vital to transmitting nerve impulses, including emotions and moods.

When SAMe made it into health and other stores, it created a storm, thanks to well-orchestrated media hype, in both print and electronic mediums, not to speak of promotional books, advertisements, and a glut of Websites. To those who adhere to the "SAMe" message, the substance is nothing short of an effective treatment for not only osteoarthritis, but also disorders like depression, and liver disease.

Studies have found 400-1,200 mg/day of SAMe as being safe. It is also free of side-effects; however, authorities caution that patients who have bipolar disorder, or Parkinson's disease, should avoid its usage.

WHAT YOU EAT IS...

What you may favour for the palate may have a role to play in the progression of osteoarthritis. This is especially found to be true if you are eating foods from the nightshade vegetable family — bell peppers, egg-plant, paprika, potatoes [excluding sweet potato and yams], and the poor man's apple, tomato. Tobacco also belongs to the nightshade family. In fact, many of the alkaloids found in nightshade plants — atropine, nicotine, and scopolamine — have been theorised to incite symptoms of [osteo]arthritis. However, the idea is not without controversy. It would, therefore, be a good idea for you to notice any "beneficial" effect/s by avoiding these plants for 6-8 weeks, if you suspect you are sensitive to them.

RIGHT DOSAGE

Researchers recommend a daily intake of 1,500 mg of glucosamine — this has been found to be appropriate for most patients. Not that you should not indulge in experimentation, and reduce your dosage. After having gone through a regimen for a period of two months, on the standard dosage, you may try taking 1,000 mg, or even something as less as 500 mg — as maintenance dose — and, see if your symptoms flare up, or you are able to keep them at bay.

Patients' and users' reports of the experimentation working to satisfaction are legion — and, so are their innumerable "miracle" stories. Whether you accept them at face value, or with some amount of unease, statistics don't lie. People, who had gone through the trauma of not having been able to move around without difficulty, have gone on record saying that their joints felt as good as they were when younger.

All the same, one point needs to be emphasised. It's always better to start early. The earlier the two supplements — glucosamine and chondroitin — are introduced into your daily nutritional plan, the better it is to prevent the disease process from getting entrenched — and, also for reversing joint damage, if any. Not that glucosamine and chondroitin will work in all individuals, but research points out that they are most likely to act best in mild-to-moderate cases of osteoarthritis, because the joints have some amount of normal and functional cartilage. The addition of glucosamine can arouse the cartilage to "kick-start" its optimal level of functioning. This may help you to most likely avoid future osteoarthritic events.

Some authorities recommend the use of either glucosamine or chondroitin, followed by a NSAID regimen, on an as-needed-basis, for better pain relief.

Studies also indicate that the reliance on NSAIDs by following such a line of treatment drops with time — in some instances, by a notable 70 per cent. The idea serves a dual purpose. By now you'd know that all that your NSAID medication does is reduce inflammation, not help you replenish healthy cartilage. So, when you reduce, if not entirely eliminate, your intake of NSAIDs, you will have decreased your risk of NSAID-related side effects, while maintaining the desired amount of inflammation, or pain, relief.

****

Chapter 9

INTEGRATIVE MEDICINE

There is a school of thought that believes in the philosophy of prescribing what suits or works best for a given individual or patient — irrespective of the fact whether it is traditional, alternative or complementary form of medicine. This body of thought opines that the use of glucosamine/chondroitin, along with the ayurvedic boswellia [Indian frankincense], may have a "synergistic" effect in the treatment of osteoarthritis. When taken together, proponents say, the two "diverse" options contribute to reducing inflammation — each in its own unique way. The net result would be a smile on the patient's face.

There are others that advocate the use of glucosamine and chondroitin alone — and, without the use of NSAIDs. They say that this form of realistically holistic treatment not only helps patients to avoid the inevitable side-effects of NSAIDs, but also eliminate their use. Some also say that a "balanced" approach would be better — increased trust on the two supplements and reduced "dependence" on NSAIDs.

ENDURING COMFORT

If you think that you have hit the Holy Grail of osteoarthritic treatment, with glucosamine and chondroitin, think again. Also, if you anticipate quick relief, or instant *nirvana*, from pain.

Research has confirmed that it takes at least a month's time for obvious benefits, with either supplement, to be experienced. The thing to look out for is continued pain relief and/or increased mobility during the first month. Most patients report that they continue to improve further in the subsequent weeks and months.

Some therapists suggest that a cyclical dosage pattern would also be fine — they say that it won't do you any harm if you taper the dose, or even reduce it [500 mg-1,000 mg], after having reached the height of your pain relief. Alternatively, they add, you may even consider not taking the supplements for a while, because the benefits don't stop the moment you do away with them.

Joint pain relief, it has also been observed, lasts for ten weeks or more, after cessation of supplement treatment. Some enterprising patients have also found that they are able to save the burden on their wallet; they just avoid the "practice" of the two-supplement daily-dose pill rule, by following another method. They have found ease by taking the two on an alternating basis.

It may also be noted here that the use of glucosamine or chondroitin topical rub-on cream, or gel, does nobody any good. It is a waste of one's money and time. Though the cream may have proven ability in the treatment of skin affections, like poison ivy or poison oak, as far as osteoarthritis is concerned, there is nothing that comes close to the oral [two-supplements] capsule/tablet.

Agreed that glucosamine and chondroitin take time to work, but it is well worth the wait — not just because those that wait never fail, but also because the analogy could be closely related to the hare and tortoise fable. Slow and steady wins the race — and, in this case, without the unwanted, or unwelcome, side-effects of conventional treatment.

CHART YOUR OWN COURSE

How do you monitor your own feel-good-treatment plan? Here it is — derived on the basis of your own Pain Record Chart, and founded on certain parameters. You'd maintain it as a register, or journal entry — a daily account of your pain, its intensity, or reduction against dates of any given month, with Pain Levels, as given below:

0 No relief

1 Mild relief

2 Moderate relief

3 Apparent relief

4 Moderately severe

5 Severe

PRECAUTIONS

Though glucosamine and chondroitin have been found to be safe for long-term use, experts recommend the following precautions to be taken before you decide on the two-supplement treatment plan.

- A significant allergy to seafood, because glucosamine [supplement] is made from chitin, found in crab, shellfish, or oyster shells [and, shark cartilage], which doesn't usually cause an allergic reaction. However, it is better to be safe than sorry

- High doses of glucosamine given intravenously to animals induce glucose intolerance. Although this has not been observed in humans, it's useful to check with your physician/therapist and/or monitor your blood sugar, if you take it. So, there it is: diabetics need not worry, but it would be better to exert extra care and precaution while taking the supplement

- If you are taking a blood-thinning medication, or daily aspirin, or have prostate affections, especially cancer, you need to exercise caution when taking chondroitin. Chondroitin is molecularly similar to the anti-coagulant, or blood thinning, properties of heparin

- Glucosamine has a slower onset than an anti-inflammatory drug, so it may take a minimum of 3-4 weeks for it to work. So, you ought to exercise patience

- Seek medical attention/opinion if you feel something is amiss; or, you have missed a dose.

You may also want to keep a watch on some of the most unlikely, or occasional, side-effects of glucosamine, in certain individuals, viz., constipation, diarrhoea, epigastric vomiting, nausea, palpitation, loss of appetite, and headache. As far as chondroitin is concerned, unlikely, or rare, side effects may include allergic reaction, with breathing difficulty, puffiness of lips, tongue, or face, and skin rash. Manageable problems all.

CONVENTIONAL TREATMENT OF OSTEOARTHRITIS

Some of the conventional medications used to treat osteoarthritis include:

Traditional pain relievers

The American College of Rheumatology recommends acetaminophen as first-line therapy for osteoarthritis. Acetaminophen is effective pain relief for many patients with osteoarthritis, because aspirin and medications such as ibuprofen are known to cause severe gastro-intestinal bleeding. Acetaminophen should be taken at a dose of 1,000 mg, 3-4 times per day. While low doses of the drug are often ineffective, high doses can cause liver damage. Also, the intake of alcohol, while taking acetaminophen, increases the risk of liver damage. Effective pain relief from the use of acetaminophen may take as long as a fortnight.

Steroid injections

As is quite well known, traditional treatments for chronic joint pain have included injections of cortisone, or other steroids, into the joint spaces. These treatments can provide lasting pain relief for several weeks. One French study evaluated 98 patients with osteoarthritis of the knee. Some received injections of steroids. Others received lavage, or washings of the joint space with sterile fluid — both groups had reduced pain for the first month. However, the patients on lavage felt better for as long as six months. The problem with steroids is their "generous" side effects.

Topical medication

NSAIDs in the form of creams and ointments offer some relief from pain when rubbed over joints. As may be quite well-known, absorption of the drug/s through the skin and into the bloodstream is theoretically possible. Hence, the fact that topical application is no guarantee that they will not cause gastro-intestinal bleeding, or kidney damage. Studies have, so far, not shown external applications to offer better benefits over oral NSAIDs, or other topical agents.

Non-steroidal anti-inflammatory drugs [NSAIDs]

Non-steroidal anti-inflammatory drugs are not discerning. They inhibit inflammatory proteins but they cannot distinguish between useful and damaging inflammatory proteins. Though they can inhibit the proteins released during inflammation that would prevent ulcers and gastro-intestinal bleeding, NSAIDs do have potentially dangerous and adverse long-term side effects. They are effective and can be used, particularly for short-term treatments, with excellent results. However, when they are prescribed for long-term use, the rule of the thumb is to prescribe an anti-ulcer medication to reduce the possibility of gastro-intestinal bleeding.

COX-2 inhibitors

Cyclooxeganase-2 [COX-2] is one of the most important proteins in our body's inflammatory response. Products from COX-2 enhance inflammation and produce pain. COX-1, a close relative, is a helpful enzyme that protects the stomach and other organs.

Traditional anti-inflammatory drugs like NSAIDs are not selective and, therefore, inhibit the action of both COX-1 and COX-2. In spite of NSAIDs' utility in the treatment of osteoarthritic pain, they also cause serious adverse effects, such as gastro-intestinal bleeding — a symptom which may be directly linked to their inhibition of COX-1.

Three new, selective COX-2 inhibitors in use have caused controversy. Refecoxib [Vioxx], celecoxib [Celebrex], and valdecoxib [Bextra]. Although studies have shown that few patients develop gastro-intestinal bleeding, doctors recommend caution in their use, particularly among the elderly. It's still early days, because the three drugs have not been in use long enough to estimate their effects on the kidneys — more so, in the developing world. Experts also favour prudence in their use with other medications — their metabolism can cause the blood levels with certain other drugs to rise to potentially perilous levels.

Besides, studies also indicate that COX-2 inhibitors have a possible connection to heart problems. They have also been thought of to cause a small increase in heart attacks and strokes —an activity that could be related to the drugs' tendency to promoting blood clots.
So, is it not better for one not to put their hearts at risk, when there are much safer, effective, and also economical, alternatives like glucosamine and chondroitin sulphate available?

Hyaluronic acid

Hyaluronic acid is another potentially valuable treatment for osteoarthritis. Hyaluronic acid is a normal component of joint cartilage; injecting it causes few adverse effects. In one limited study conducted at the University of Cincinnati, US, 61 patients with osteoarthritis — of one or both knees — received three weekly injections of hyaluronic acid into their painful knees. A vast majority of the patients experienced relief of pain and improvement in function that lasted up to 24 weeks after the completion of treatment.

In another large study conducted in Indianapolis, US, 226 patients with osteoarthritis of the knee were assessed to ascertain the efficacy of injected hyaluronic acid. In a report published in *Clinical Orthopaedics*, the investigators surmised that 58 per cent of patients, who received injections of hyaluronic acid, experienced an improvement in their pain levels, as compared to only 40 per cent of those who had received injections of only salt water [saline].

Surgery

Surgery often plays its part in the treatment of severe osteoarthritis, especially in patients who do not get pain relief from medication, home treatment, or other methods, and who have had significant loss of cartilage. Surgical intervention relieves severe, disabling pain and may also restore joint function and mobility. Some surgical procedures, such as osteotomy or arthroscopy, may be done to postpone total joint replacement.

The surgical options include:

- *Arthroscopy.* This can provide temporary and also long-term relief of symptoms of osteoarthritis. It may also be used to fix a joint, if it becomes "locked," or stuck, due to loose cartilage or bone fragments.
- *Osteotomy of the knee and the hip.* This is used in cases of hip deformity and abnormality of the legs in active people [<60] with mild osteoarthritis
- *Knee replacement surgery.* This is considered in cases of knee pain associated with disability and damage that is visible on X-rays.

- *Hip replacement surgery.* This is considered in cases of pain accompanied by disability and deterioration of the hip visible on X-rays.

- *Arthrodesis.* This surgery helps join [fuse] two bones in a diseased joint, or when the joint can no longer move. It may be used for the spine, ankles, hands, and feet. However, the procedure is rarely used in weight-bearing joints [knees and hips].

- *Small joint replacement surgery.* This is used if the joints of the hands are so disabled that function is almost out of question. [*Note:* The severity of finger disability is more common in rheumatoid arthritis, and not so much in osteoarthritis. Read also, page 101].

Surgery is not a cure for osteoarthritis. It is also very expensive. Besides this, the artificial joint has a lifespan of about 10 years, and surgery will have to be repeated again. This, of course, excludes those cases of cementless hip replacements, where bone and metal fuse have been performed.

Quantum Magnetic Resonance Therapy

Quantum Magnetic Resonance Therapy [QMR Therapy™] method is suggested to be a painless, safe, non-invasive and cost-effective alternative method of treatment when compared to surgery. Proponents surmise that it is the world's first "scientifically" proven, non-surgical treatment to help build cartilage and restore mobility of arthritic knee joints.

****

Chapter 10

ALTERNATIVE THERAPIES

Transcutaneous electrical nerve stimulation

This treatment, also abbreviated TENS, is often used by conventional physical therapists. In one study of 78 patients with osteoarthritis of the knee, TENS has shown some benefit in reducing pain and increasing function. Also, physical therapy can improve physical functioning and limit pain by strengthening and stabilising joints.

Used in conjunction with conventional treatment, physical therapy can help patients achieve effective relief and minimise future decline in joint health.

Magnet therapy

A host of studies on animal bone and cartilage in the laboratory has shown that pulsing magnetic fields leads to an improvement in bone [fracture] healing time and cartilage cell growth. However, no long-term controlled studies have been done that demonstrate the effectiveness of this treatment.

Therapeutic touch

Some call it mumbo-jumbo: some faith healing. In this form of treatment, the hands of the practitioner are held above the part of the body to be treated. In one study of 25 patients with osteoarthritis of the knee, therapeutic touch showed that people who were treated with it experienced statistically significant improvement in pain and function. Larger studies are wanting; they need to be conducted to confirm the method's efficacy, if any.

Acupuncture

Acupuncture has given conflicting results; some studies showing good relief from pain: some showing no benefit at all.

A study on 73 patients conducted at the University of Maryland School of Medicine, US, compared acupuncture to standard care for osteoarthritis; those who received acupuncture showed improvements in a span of 1-2 months. However, the improvement tended to decline after 12 weeks. More studies would be needed to confirm the benefits of acupuncture in the treatment of osteoarthritis.

Yoga

The ancient Indian system of yoga offers at least hypothetical benefits for osteoarthritic patients. Indeed, trials have shown subjective improvement in pain for those with osteoarthritis of the hands. Further study of this treatment is also warranted, although it is a proven fact that yoga involves stretching and strengthening that heals the body and its joints.

Diathermy

Deep heat, or diathermy, has been reported as a valuable aid for controlling pain and joint mobility. The treatment is administered by ultrasound [high frequency sound waves], or microwave [electromechanical irradiation], or short wave.

Diathermy works on the principle that application of heat is thought to increase the pain threshold and ameliorate pain by reducing nerve-conduction velocity. The only drawback — diathermy is not only uneconomical for patients, but it is also a long drawn-out, time-consuming process.

Leeches

Don't you think that we are going back to mediaeval times! This is one fact that "proves" that not everything old isn't good. A group of investigators found that leeches could reduce the pain and inflammation of osteoarthritis of the knee.

Ten patients were treated with topical application of four leeches to their osteoarthritis knees, for 80 minutes. They experienced a significant reduction in pain within 24 hours. These results lasted for as long as four weeks. Patients also experienced no side-effects or infection.

Researchers contemplate that leech saliva contains compounds that relieve pain, by causing actual anaesthesia to the joints, and reducing inflammation. Larger trials are recommended before conclusions are made.

Other forms of alternative therapy include occupational therapy using assisted devices to fit your circumstance, massage therapy, or its Japanese corollary [shiatsu], chiropractic [manipulation of bones and joints], homeopathy, cognitive/behavioural therapy, and relaxation techniques like meditation.

Homeopathy

Homeopathic remedies have been praised in the treatment of osteoarthritis. Here is an outline.

Bryonia alba: Joints violently inflamed, swollen, red, shiny and extremely "hot." Aggravation from slightest motion, touch and pressure.

Colchicum autumnale: Affections of the joints, fingers, toes, wrists and ankles. Violent pains. The patient cannot bear to have the parts touched. Movement aggravates. General symptoms of profound weakness and gastric derangement.

Guaiacum officinale: A great remedy in chronic osteoarthritis. Tendons contracted. Limbs drawn out of shape. Immovable stiffness. Gout.

Ledum palustre: One of the best remedies, especially in sub-acute osteoarthritis. Nodes form in joints. Arthritic pains that travel upwards; worse by warmth. Ankles and big toe swollen. Gouty inflammations.

Picric acid and *Urtica urens*: Are said to be most useful in obstinate cases.

Other useful homeopathic medicines are *Causticum Hahnemanni, Rhus toxicodendron,* and *Silicea terra* [especially in familial osteoarthritis].

A combination of alternative therapies, along with conventional/supplemental treatment, experts say, may be most desirable and useful when well-chosen treatments fail to give results.

BEYOND ARTHRITIS

While researchers are focused on using their compass and radar on the two supplements' — glucosamine and chondroitin — proven attributes in dealing with osteoarthritis, there are several other benefits that have accrued by their use. Did you know that the duo, for example, has the ability to reduce your cholesterol levels and also help you stop snoring? There are other benefits too, and let us summarise them — so that you expand on the overall benefits you'd derive from their use.

Therosclerosis

Heart diseases claim millions of lives each year — more than any other disease. Though the progression of cardiovascular disease is complex, elevated cholesterol levels are closely linked to the development of atherosclerosis — hardening of the arteries. As a result, the walls of the arteries lose their elasticity. This impedes proper circulation. It also leads to the build-up of fatty deposits. In atherosclerosis, the arteries are not only hard; they are inflexible. Clogged with clusters of cholesterol, they are more likely to develop high blood pressure. When the coronary arteries [blood vessels that feed the heart], get clogged, it leads to coronary artery disease. The stage is set for a heart attack.

Studies have demonstrated the efficacy of chondroitin sulphate in protecting the health of blood vessels in the heart. Chondroitin lines the blood vessels and prevents the clumping of platelets. It also lowers blood cholesterol levels. So, if you are taking chondroitin for your aching joints, would it not be heartening to know that you are also providing some healthy benefits to your heart?

Kidney stone and other conditions

Kidney stones are formed when substances in the urine — like oxalate — precipitate into stones. They can cause severe pain, accompanied by chills, fever, and nausea. Calcium stone is the more common type of kidney stone. Because, chondroitin is naturally present in the urinary system, lining the bladder wall, researchers report that it can help lower urinary oxalate levels in individuals prone to accumulating oxalates.

Chondroitin sulphate may also be used in conditions such as dry eyes [Sjögren's syndrome] — where your tear ducts don't make enough tears. Dry eyes are common in women, especially after menopause; it can also be suggestive of a serious health problem, such as RA, lupus [varying degree of pain in joints, with redness and swelling], or side-effects of medical treatment.

Research has shown that the inclusion of chondroitin in artificial tear products can help dry eyes patients improve their ability to reduce burning, itching, and that typical feeling of a foreign body in the eye, which is common in the condition.

Other disorders where chondroitin sulphate has been found useful are migraine, snoring [chondroitin forms a coating on the nasal passages and curbs your "Nosey Master's Noise"], and temporomandibular joint syndrome [TMJ], a disorder of the upper jaw.

Glucosamine and chondroitin are also useful in stomach ulcers, because the former stimulates the production of protective gastric mucous — and boosts the stomach's resistance to ulcers. This is not all. Perfect raw materials for replacement skin and other soft tissues, the two supplements have it in them to promote wound healing too.

GET YOUR DOCTOR TO KNOW

Though a prescription is not needed for you to buy the two dietary supplements — and/or vitamins, minerals, SAMe etc., — it would be a good idea for you to seek the opinion of your doctor before treating your osteoarthritis symptoms with them. This would guarantee that you are in no doubt, thanks to your doctor's expert opinion, that the source of your joint problems is osteoarthritis, not bursitis, gout, lupus, or RA.

****

CONCLUSION

Osteoarthritis can be a debilitating disease with significant long-term costs of treatment. Costs include not only the tangible expense for therapies, but also loss of productivity at the workplace. While weight reduction, exercise and physical therapy, have been found to be useful in many patients, most therapeutic strategists consider NSAIDs as their first-line of pharmacotherapeutic approach, or line of treatment.

One major worry is NSAIDs, and other conventional drugs, have been associated with a host of dangerous and adverse side-effects that can also sometimes limit their utility in some patients. Aside from this, NSAIDs do not provide the means to transform the disease process. Instead, they confine themselves to treat the symptoms of pain.

Glucosamine and chondroitin have been investigated for their ability to alter underlying cartilage "erosion." The inference: they provide potential pain relief in osteoarthritis.

Also, a vast majority of studies in medical literature has demonstrated the ability of glucosamine sulphate to allaying osteoarthritic symptoms in a manner that is quite superior to placebo and, at least, equally effective to NSAIDs, such as ibuprofen, but without their side-effects.

Furthermore, the side-effect profile of glucosamine sulphate also appears quite insignificant in comparison to NSAIDs.

Also, a number of resourceful clinical trials are being published in literature, from time to time, that clearly support the use of glucosamine sulphate/chondroitin sulphate in the treatment of osteoarthritis.

New reports suggest that a combination of glucosamine sulphate and chondroitin sulphate may be even more efficacious in the treatment of osteoarthritis — this, of course, complemented by long-term pain relief and comfort.

The conclusion is evident. If dietary, nutritional supplements provide us a dependable tool-kit, without causing us any harm, why don't you try them out? Enter, glucosamine and chondroitin — more so, in the light of the fact that NSAIDs, and other drugs, cause more harm than good, a documented fact.

From the time the great nineteenth century British physician, Sir William Osler, came up with his famous metaphor, or despair, for not having a workable treatment for joint agony — "When an arthritis patient walks in the front door, I feel like leaving by the back door" — not much has changed in the conventional school of medicine.

Not that researchers aren't trying hard — they sure are doing their best and more. However, all their good work seems to be rendered deficient in view of every new, or new-found already-in-use, drug's side-effect profile.

Isn't it ironic that in the background of high-tech research, and in this age of amazing scientific advance, we now find two unpretentious, but quite celebrated, natural and nutritional supplements, promising us hope — a quiet, efficient method of doing what conventional physicians cannot do?

A sure, safe way to relieving joint inflammation, immobility, and the agony of osteoarthritis — while, at the same time, promoting the growth of new, healthy cartilage!

Not only this. Isn't it also time, therefore, that you gave them a good shot, a fair trial, and an opportunity to work on you — so that your joints get the shine back into their life, and your life, too?

****

Beat Osteoarthritis, Naturally

Arthritis is a degenerative disorder of the joints, characterised by pain and inflammation.

The most common form of arthritic affection, osteoarthritis [OA], affects millions of people worldwide — as a matter of fact, it seems to be more common than heart ailments and diabetes.

Call it an irony, or what you may, one major fact remains — osteoarthritis is only going to expand in its intensity, and also get firmly rooted in one's middle years, sooner than later.

Experts estimate that over three million people visit their doctor for osteoarthritis, in the UK, every year. It affects millions of people in India too, aside from over 20 million in the US.

Osteoarthritis is characterised by loss of cartilage and joint degeneration. It is a condition that is much more common in men at age 45; it becomes more predominant in women over age 45.

Osteoarthritis, to put it mildly, robs you of your basic ability to get fully engaged in day-to-day activity. In its early stages, it may affect one joint, or multiple joints; besides, it varies in its intensity, or severity.

Needless to say, osteoarthritis is one of man's oldest afflictions.

OA is a chronic disease; its name is derived from Greek: "osteo," refers to bones; "orthro," to joints involved; and, "itis," referring to the inflammatory process of the disease.

It is estimated that Americans alone spend over $15 billion a year in an attempt to alleviate arthritis pain. Add to this, the expenditure on arthritis medicines worldwide, and you have a huge market, nay an industry, catering to patients' needs.

NSAIDs: Damaging side-effects

One of the most conventional modes of treatment to ease arthritis pain is the use of prescription drugs — non-steroidal anti-inflammatory drugs [NSAIDs], which are quite expensive. Furthermore, the long-term use of these medications is known to lead to dangerous side-effects.

Reports estimate that thousands of patients suffer from gastro-intestinal bleeding as a direct result of NSAID use, every year. Ironically, though these drugs are used for arthritis pain relief, they are known to actually hasten the destruction of cartilage itself. One study, conducted in Norway, has found that OA patients taking Indocin, a strong NSAID, had far more rapid destruction of the hip than the group not taking any NSAID.

The Journal of the American Medical Association [JAMA], to underline the point, reports severe liver damage caused by Voltaren, a NSAID most frequently prescribed for arthritis in the US. The journal also reports that patients developed hepatitis within 4-6 weeks of taking the medication, and also possible liver damage, weeks after taking the drug.

Steroids ain't good

Corticosteroids, like NSAIDs, are also used to control inflammation and suppress symptoms. They seem to have just as many bad effects as NSAIDs; perhaps, more.

According to the noted alternative physician, Dr Julian Whitaker, "These agents [corticosteroids] are so powerful that, even at lower doses, a handful of side-effects are not just possible, they are expected. On less than 10 mg per day, an individual will feel increased appetite. Salt and water will be retained. The individual will gain weight. And, the person will get sick more often. Research shows an increased susceptibility to infections in [rheumatoid] arthritis patients on corticosteroids..."

Whitaker elaborates: "If the dose is stepped up, a whole cascade of problems can emerge. There are cosmetic problems, such as acne and increasing facial hair in women. Individuals may begin to feel muscle cramps and weakness. The individual's skin may thin and weaken. Peptic ulcers may develop. Blood pressure may rise, with its attendant risks. Diabetes can develop. So can osteoporosis. Susceptibility to blood clot formation increases. It is suggested that over one half [57 per cent] of individuals on corticosteroids have depression, or other mental, or emotional disturbances. This is not surprising, considering the onslaught of side-effects overlaid on their original disease."

What next?

When NSAIDs and steroids stop to halt the progression of arthritis, patients are often asked to switch over to a third option, down the line — this drug therapy consists of methotrexate, cyclophosphamide, penicillamine.

Also, Hydroxychloroquine, azathioprine, and gold therapy. They are, in essence, toxic disease-modifying drugs, which are administered concurrently with NSAIDs and corticosteroids.

According to a study published in *The Lancet*, which looked at 112 patients who were on such aggressive drug therapy over a 20-year period, over one-third [35 per cent] had died and another fifth [19 per cent] were severely disabled. Most of the mortality and morbidity, the study pointed out, was directly related to rheumatoid arthritis and its treatment. Interestingly, the study observed that only 18 per cent of patients were able to lead normal lives.

Wait a moment. There are, in addition, anti-inflammatories such as anacin, aspirin, and acetaminophen [paracetamol] that can lead to serious, unfavourable effects. It is estimated that almost 15-20 per cent individuals/patients who take large doses of these non-prescription, or OTC, drugs are likely to develop serious gastric ulcers.

In the US alone, it is estimated that 15,000 of them die from gastro-intestinal haemorrhages, every year.

It is also said that kidney failure is another possible side-effect of NSAIDs, especially in individuals whose blood flow is inadequate, owing to age and/or on account of medications.

The big question

Now, the big question — what happens when drugs, like NSAIDs or steroids, no longer help you?

You are witness to the most likely scenario. Your doctor will hurl his/her hands up in the air, with a touch of disgust, and say, "There's nothing much we can do for you, apart from surgery!"

So, you move on to the next step — with hope and also apprehension.

Arthritis surgery often consists of one or more of the following procedures:

- Synovectomy, or removal of badly inflamed joint synovium
- Anthroplasty, or joint realignment and reconstruction
- Joint fusion, or tendon repair
- Artificial joint replacement, in the most severe cases, which is also the most expensive, and extremely profitable for the one performing the procedure. It is also the most painful of surgical procedures with protracted recovery time and recuperation.

It is estimated that 50 per of joint replacement patients continue to have pain and restricted mobility following the operation. Many also experience extreme discomfort than before the surgery. Patients, who manage to get through, tend to often have problems with the operated joint three-four years later, and may require to undergo the procedure again in 8-10 years. Add to this the cause of the joint problems having not been corrected, and you will probably come back with the disorder in other parts of the body. You will have nothing but only regret, thereafter.

Hence, the big question — if existing drugs and medical procedures don't work, is there anything else, which is useful and free from deleterious side-effects, the arthritis sufferer can resort to, for relief?

Nature nurtures

Thank nature for big mercies! This is not all. New research is throwing fresh light on natural remedies and opening up new treatment avenues for relief from arthritic agony.

Let's look at some of the natural arthritis remedies, or supplements, also called nutraceuticals, that natural physicians/therapists recommend the most. These remedies are all well-documented and have proven effective in the treatment of osteoarthritis.

Glucosamine sulphate

The most widely used natural substance for osteoarthritis, glucosamine offers a low-cost and safe alternative to arthritis drugs. Besides this, it provides, in most cases, better pain relief than prescription, or over-the-counter [OTC], medication.

Several studies have found that by adding glucosamine, a naturally occurring substance in our body, back to the body in supplement form, leads to enhanced connective tissue healing and regeneration.

Glucosamine has been a boon for anyone suffering from diseases related to cartilage destruction. It may also be further said that glucosamine treats the root cause of the problem rather than just suppressing the symptoms as do standard drug therapies. In addition, glucosamine, unlike NSAIDs, is considered safe and non-toxic. The best part — it can be used for extended periods of time without any hazard.

Chondroitin sulphate

When glucosamine is combined with chondroitin sulphate, another naturally-occurring substance in the body, it has been found to be extremely effective in treating osteoarthritis. Several research studies also evidence the effectiveness of this combination as a safe and effective arthritis treatment plan. Glucosamine and chondroitin, which are both popular supplements of choice today, work together synergistically to initiate the production of new cartilage. At the same time, they protect the existing cartilage tissue, and prevent damage to it.

Glucosamine and chondroitin have received wide acceptance after the mid-1990s.

In addition, the following natural substances, according to latest research studies, have also been shown to reduce the symptoms of OA.

Cetyl myristoleate [CMO]

CMO is a natural immuno-modulator. It is believed to help regulate and normalise a faulty immune system, and reduce or impede the arthritic process itself. It works on nature's own premise — that once joint deterioration stops, and pain and inflammation are relieved, the body can heal itself from within and return to normalcy.

First discovered by Harry W Diehl, while working alone in his home laboratory, CMO is essentially oil. It has sure come a long way...

While a host of published research reports commend its positive value in relieving joint pain, some studies have also corroborated its use to "modulate the inflammatory process" — the hub of your arthritic agony.

Here's testimony:

- In a double-blind study, which included 64 patients, with chronic osteoarthritis [OA] of the knee joint, half of the patients received a CMO complex; the other half received a placebo, or dummy pill. Measurements included physician review, assessment of knee joint function, and the Lequesne Index — a research tool used to measure the severity of OA symptoms. The result? Patients in the CMO group showed significant improvement, while patients in the placebo group showed little or no improvement. Researchers in the study concluded that CMO "may be an alternative to the use of non-steroidal anti-inflammatory drugs [NSAIDs] for the treatment of OA." — *The Journal of Rheumatology*

- In another study that included 1,814 arthritis patients, results showed that over 87 per cent of the subjects had greater than 50 per cent recovery, and over 65 per cent showed 75 per cent to 100 per cent recovery, following a 16-day treatment on CMO. — *Advanced Medical Systems & Design, Ltd.,*

This is not all. Says Dr Douglas Hunt, who was one among the first medical pioneers to research and study the long- and short-term effects of cetyl myristoleate: "CMO does its job! Many who have taken CMO have been free of joint and muscle pain for as long as nine years."

Studies have also found that when CMO is combined with sea cucumber — a natural anti-inflammatory agent — the "shared" formula is rendered more effective and potent to relieve arthritic pain from its roots.

Sea cucumber, which has a long history of medicinal use in the Orient, encompasses a nerve-blocking agent — holothurin. Holothurin has been stated to relieve joint pain and stiffness — naturally. Besides, research also confirms the fact that sea cucumber is useful for many inflammatory conditions — not just osteoarthritis and rheumatoid arthritis, but also ankylosing spondylitis, and so on.

Sea cucumber, studies further report, has the ability to balance prostaglandins, which regulate the inflammatory process. Besides, it contains both chondroitin and mucopolysaccharides, which are "undersupplied" in arthritic patients. When the two elements are incorporated in your medicinal/treatment regimen, they not only reduce inflammation, but also help in tissue repair and lubrication of your joints.

MSM [Methylsulphonylmethane]

MSM is a natural sulphur compound. It is also one of the most important compounds found in our body. It is just as essential as water and sodium.

Our MSM levels reduce with age. This results in symptoms of fatigue, tissue and organ malfunction; also, increased vulnerability to illness. One study found almost 80 per cent control of joint pain within the first six weeks of treatment with MSM.

The combined use of glucosamine and MSM for symptomatic pain relief and tissue repair in joints is preferred in some of the scientific literature today; also, side-effects, even if they occur, are often mild in nature and controllable.

SAMe [S-adenosylmethionine]

SAMe [S-adenosylmethionine], like MSM, is also a natural product that has been proven to offer therapeutic benefits in osteoarthritis. In addition, it appears to promote production of cartilage proteoglycans, and is, therefore, beneficial in osteoarthritis in well-controlled oral doses. Needless to say, SAMe and/or other safe nutritional measures, which support proteoglycans synthesis, may offer a practical means of preventing or delaying the onset of osteoarthritis in older individuals or athletes.

Other useful natural remedies

Boswellia has been used for centuries in ayurveda, the ancient Indian system of medicine, to maintain healthy joints. It inhibits inflammation, decreases cartilage synthesis, improves blood supply to the joints and maintains the integrity of blood vessels.

Vitamin C is said to protect and enhance cartilage formation. High intake of vitamin C, a powerful anti-oxidant, has also been suggested to reduce the risk of cartilage loss and slow down the progression of osteoarthritis.

Vitamin E is another powerful anti-oxidant that protects the joints from free radical damage and increases joint mobility.

Essential fatty acids [EFA] are necessary to produce substances that lubricate the joints. The most important is EFA [omega-3], found in cold water fish, flaxseed, and other food sources.

Some authorities also recommend the use of vitamin B5 and B6, zinc, copper and boron for the manufacture and maintenance of normal cartilage structure. A deficiency of any one of these nutrients is suggested to hasten joint degeneration.

Efficient, but not instant

These natural products, though usefully effective, are not quick-fixes or cures. You'd first need to realise that inflammation must be stopped and the tissue rebuilt before OA pain can come to a standstill — completely.

Also, the elder or older the person is, the longer the rebuilding process. However, while some people notice results in a week or two after using natural remedies, a clear-cut difference should be felt after about six weeks. Make sure, however, that you use good quality natural arthritis products combined with appropriate lifestyle modifications. This can really speed up the curative process.

One thing you would do well to bear in mind is — the damage to the joints didn't happen suddenly. It was a slow process. Hence, its repair will also take time. Once this happens, you and your joints will be all the more contented for it.

****

Appendix

Facts You Should Know

All of us go through the "grind" of daily life — call it wear and tear, or what you may. The fact is not all of us, despite our best intentions, eat a perfect diet. What's more, we are all prone to minor mishaps — a fall, or a sports injury. Besides, all of us need to face the inevitable — the process of aging. All of these, and more, can lead to damaged cartilage, ligaments, and tendons.

To lead a life of optimal well-being, we need to eat a balanced diet and exercise to keep our joints healthy. This is fundamental to staying active and living a "pain-free" life. Glucosamine and chondroitin help to keep and/or maintain our joints resilient and strong. The duo achieves this prospect by lubricating and repairing our connective tissues — from the so-called wear and tear of day-to-day life.

Synonyms

Glucosamine sulphate; glucosamine hydrochloride [HCl]

Chondroitin sulphate

Availability

You don't get the duo in everyday foods. You need to obtain them from supplements derived from shellfish, albeit you now have vegan glucosamine derived from fermented corn.

Key role

Glucosamine and chondroitin strengthen the connective tissues [cartilage, ligaments, and tendons]; they keep them healthy and supple.

The duo helps regenerate damaged cartilage — this helps restore joint function, aside from mobility. It also helps to promote recovery from injury in quick time.

Deficiency

There is no question of deficiency; the fact is steady, repeated use and strain on particular joints and tendons, caused by weight training and sporting activities, often produce the "overuse" syndrome. This may sometimes lead to depletion of healthy connective tissue.

Research

Research indicates that the duo could be useful in the treatment of:

- Osteoarthritis

- Wounds/injuries

- Connective tissue disorders

- Bone and joint problems

Dosage

Glucosamine, 1,500 mg; chondroitin, 800 mg, daily.

Timing

Preferably, with meals.

Role of vitamin C

The duo seems to work synergistically with vitamin C; this also helps the body to produce and stabilise healthy collagen in the connective tissues.

Toxicity

There is no known toxicity.

Restrictions

None reported yet.

Fact-File

What are glucosamine and chondroitin?

Glucosamine is the precursor to a molecule called glycosaminoglycan; this molecule is used in the formation and repair of cartilage.

Chondroitin is the most plentiful glycosaminoglycan in cartilage; it is responsible for the elasticity of cartilage.

Do glucosamine and chondroitin supplements really increase cartilage formation?

Though purists do not fancy the idea, clinical studies have shown that the consumption of the two joint supplements increases the quantity of cartilage building blocks within a joint.

What studies report about glucosamine and chondroitin?

There have been numerous studies to examine the therapeutic effects and benefits of glucosamine and chondroitin. There are also evidence-based studies showing definitive pain reduction in individuals taking glucosamine and chondroitin than patients receiving placebo [dummy pill]. The improvement experienced is suggested to be similar to improvement experienced by patients on NSAIDs — the mainstay of non-operative conventional arthritis treatment. NSAIDs, of course, carry an increased risk of side-effects, including gastro-intestinal bleeding.

The best part: glucosamine and chondroitin have just a few, minor side-effects, if any.

It is also suggested that NSAIDs may increase the progression of osteoarthritis — instead of easing pain in the joints, for which they are given. On the other hand, glucosamine and chondroitin are suggested to offer a protective outcome to cartilage.

Who uses glucosamine the most?

People who are physically active. Sportspersons. Because, years of repetitive motion and/or overuse of joints may lead to cartilage damage? Yes. This is often presented by way of aching shoulders, knees, and elbows. Also, the elderly age group, or seniors, more so when they begin to present with symptoms and signs of osteoarthritis. When there is major cartilage damage, it leads to friction on the bone at the joints. In course of time, this may make things difficult for natural movement. Studies show that glucosamine and chondroitin help combat the condition by regenerating cartilage and/or stimulating the production of connective tissue.

Should I take glucosamine or chondroitin, or both?

Glucosamine and chondroitin are evidenced to stimulate the joint cells to produce better quality synovial fluid, which acts as a cushion. The two also prompt the cartilage matrix to help prevent damage to the joints.

When key, or refined, isolates of the two supplements are taken, they are easily absorbed in the bloodstream. They sift easily through the capillaries to their proposed goal — the joints. Once this happens, they trigger the body to produce its own natural glucosamine and chondroitin.

How do the two supplements work?

Molecules from the two supplements journey in the bloodstream to the soft tissues of the joint. Glucosamine and chondroitin are produced naturally in the body. They are the building blocks for cartilage and act as a cushion-pad for joint fluid.

Can one take the two supplements as preventative therapy?

Yes. Anyone can take them as joint supplements for natural joint health. Remember, they are not medicines. For those who wish to maintain a life of optimal health and well-being, they are what the natural therapist ordered.

Can one take glucosamine and chondroitin, along with other medications?

Although the two supplements have no known side-effects, it is always better to speak to your physician/therapist, if you have any concerns about prescription medicines that you may be already taking. Experts suggest the use of glucosamine with vitamin C, bromelain, chondroitin sulphate, or manganese, may actually augment the therapeutic benefits for osteoarthritis.

It's also evidenced that there may be an added benefit in individuals suffering from psoriasis, especially when glucosamine is taken with fish oil.

I have a known allergy. Can I take the two supplements?

Individuals who are allergic to shellfish would do well to speak to their physician/therapist before taking the supplements.

Where should I buy my supplements?

It is recommended that you buy your supplements manufactured by reputed companies and from good health food stores.

What are the most common side-effects of the two supplements?

- Bloating; gas

- Soft stools

- Stomach upset

- Sleepiness

- Sleeplessness

- Headache

- Skin reaction

- Sun sensitivity

- Toughened nails

- Marginal rise of blood pressure and heart rate, in some individuals.

Do the two supplements affect blood sugar levels?

Individuals who have low blood sugar are advised to be careful when taking glucosamine. It may be a good idea for them to have blood sugar levels monitored frequently. Speak to your physician/therapist, if you have concerns, or other health problems.

Can glucosamine and chondroitin increase the risk of bleeding like NSAIDs?

Individuals on blood-thinning medications, or a daily aspirin, should monitor their blood clotting time frequently. Your supplement dosages need to be altered, if there is any major change — this can be done in consultation with your physician/therapist.

Can the two supplements be taken during pregnancy and/or breastfeeding?

It is strongly recommended that glucosamine be avoided during pregnancy and breastfeeding. They are also not recommended for use in children.

Endnote

Whether you suffer from joint pain associated with simple wear and tear, or you have an old nagging sports injury, or, perhaps, early onset of osteoarthritis, glucosamine is a intelligent choice for regenerating joint health. Because glucosamine is similar in its structural properties, as well as mechanisms of action, to chondroitin sulphate, new research has indicated that they may work more effectively, even synergistically, when used together. This is also suggested to help fight inflammation, relieve connective-tissue damage, and restore joints to good health.

References

1. Fauci, Braunwald, Wilson et al. Harrison's **Principles of Internal Medicine.** McGraw-Hill. 15th Edition.

2. Constantz R B. **Glucosamine and Chondroitin Sulfate: Roles for Therapy in Arthritis?** In: Kelley W N, Harris E D, Ruddy S, Sledge C B, Eds. Textbook of Rheumatology. W B Saunders, 1998.

3. Weatherby C, Gordin L, MD. **The Arthritis Bible.** Healing Arts Press.

4. Mindell E L. **The MSM Miracle: Enhance Your Health with Organic Sulfur.** Keats Publishing, Inc.,

5. M J Tapadinhas, I C Rivera, A A Bignamini. **Oral Glucosamine sulphate in the Management of Arthrosis: Report on a Multi-centre Open Investigation in Portugal.** Pharmacotherapeutica, 1982; 3:157-68.

6. Karel Pavelká, MD, PhD, Jindriska Gatterová, MD, Marta Olejarová, MD, Stanislav Machacek, MD, Giampaolo Giacovelli, PhD, Lucio C Rovati, MD. **Glucosamine sulfate Use and Delay of Progression of Knee Osteoarthritis: A 3-Year, Randomized, Placebo-controlled, Double-blind Study.** Arch Intern Med. 2002; 162:2113-2123.

7. Reginster J Y, Gillot V, Bruyere O, Henrotin Y. **Evidence of Nutraceutical Effectiveness in the Treatment of Osteoarthritis.** Curr Rheumatol Rep. 2000; 2:472-77.

8. Deal C L, Moskowitz R W. **Nutraceuticals as Therapeutic Agents in Osteoarthritis: The Role of Glucosamine,** Chondroitin sulfate, and Collagen hydrolysate. Rheum Dis Clin North Am. 1999; 25:379-95.

9. McAlindon T E, LaValley M P, Gulin J P, Felson D T. **Glucosamine and Chondroitin for the Treatment of Osteoarthritis: A Systematic Quality Assessment and Meta-analysis.** JAMA. 2000; 283:1469-75.

10. Reichelt et al. **Efficacy and Safety of Intramuscular Glucosamine sulfate in Osteoarthritis of the Knee.** Arzneimittelforschung. 1994; 444[1]:75-80,

11. Vaz et al. **Double-blind Clinical Evaluation of the Relative Efficacy of Ibuprofen and Glucosamine sulphate in the Management of Osteoarthritis of the Knee in Out-patients.** Curr Med Res Opin. 1982; 8[3]:145–149.

12. Noack W et al. **Glucosamine sulphate in Osteoarthritis of the Knee. Osteoarthritis and Cartilage.** 1994; 2:51-59.

13. Puljate J M et al. **Osteoarthritis and Cartilage.** 1994; 2[Suppl.1]:56.

14. D'Ambrosio E et al. Pharmatherapeutica. 1981; 2[8]:504-8.

15. Gaby A R. **Natural Treatments for Osteoarthritis.** Alt Med Rev. 1999: 4:330-341.

16. McCarthy F. **The Neglect of Glucosamine as a Treatment for Osteoarthritis.** Medi Hypotheses. 1994; 42[5]:323-27.

17. Setnikar I. **Anti-reactive Properties of Chondroprotective Drugs.** Int J Tissue React. 1992; 14[5]:253-61.

18. Morrison M. **Therapeutic Applications of Chondroitin sulphate: Appraisal of Biologic Properties.** Folia Angiol. 1977; 25:225-32.

19. Dovanti A, Bignamini A A, Rovati A L. **Therapeutic Activity of Oral Glucosamine sulphate in Osteoarthritis: A Placebo-controlled Double-blind Investigation.** Clin Ther. 1980; 3[4]:266-72.

20. Basleer C et al. **International Journal of Tissue Reaction.** 1992; 14:231.

21. Bland J H, Cooper S M. **Osteoarthritis: Evidence for Reversibility. Semin Arthritis Rheum.** 1984; 14:106-33.

22. Florent Richy, MSc, University of Liege, Belgium. **Arch of Intern Med,** July 14, 2003.

23. Srinivas L, Shalini V K, Shylaja M. Turmerin: **A Water-soluble Anti-oxidant Peptide from Turmeric.** Arch Biochem Biophys. 1992; 292[2]:617-23.

24. Nidamboor R. **Health-Prism,** 2008.

Resources

- Arthritis Research Campaign
  Tel: 0870-850-5000
  http://www.arc.org.uk

- Arthritis Care
  Tel: 0808-800-4050
  http://www.arthritiscare.org.uk

- Arthritis Foundation
  Website: www.arthritis.org

- American Pain Society
  Tel: [847] 375-4715
  Website: www.ampainsoc.org

- American Academy of Orthopaedic Surgeons
  Tel: [800] 824-BONE [2663]
  Website: www.aaos.org

- National Institute of Arthritis and Musculoskeletal and Skin
  Diseases
  Tel: [301] 565-2966
  Fax: [301] 718-6366
  Website: www.niams.nih.gov

- American College of Rheumatology
  Tel: [404] 633 3777
  Fax: [404] 633 1870
  Website: www.rheumatology.org

- Alternative Medicine Foundation, Inc.,
  Tel: [301] 340-1960
  Fax: [301] 340-1936
  http://www.amfoundation.org

- National Center for Complementary and Alternative
  Medicine [NCCAM]
  Tel: [888] 644-6226
  Fax: [866] 464-3616
  http://nccam.nih.gov

- Samved Orthopaedic Institute [India]
  http://samved-ortho.com

Glossary

- *Acupuncture.* Ancient Chinese technique that uses needles to pierce specific areas of the body along nerve pathways. Acupuncture may be used to relieve pain, induce anaesthesia, or serve as a treatment for diseases.

- *Arthrodesis.* Surgical fusion of a joint. The joint becomes stiff after the surfaces of the joint are removed and the bone ends are united.

- *Arthroscopy.* The examination of the inside of a joint using a device with a tiny video camera.

- *Cartilage.* Fibrous, flexible connective tissue that cushions the ends of the bones within the joints and serves as a framework for bone development in the foetus.

- *Chondroitin.* Chondroitin [sulphate] is a natural substance found in the body. It prevents other body enzymes from degrading the building blocks of joint cartilage.

- *Collagen.* A protein that makes up the white fibres of connective tissue, such as cartilage.

- *Corticosteroids.* Medications [e.g., prednisone] that are related to cortisone, a naturally occurring hormone. Corticosteroids lessen inflammation, swelling, and pain. In some cases, corticosteroids are injected directly into a joint; however, they can have serious side-effects — such as damage to bones and cartilage — especially when used over long periods of time.

- *COX-2 inhibitors.* A new class of medications that were developed to manage the symptoms of arthritis without negative gastro-intestinal effects. COX-2 inhibitors stop the activity of specific cyclooxygenase [COX] enzymes, which release prostaglandins [responsible for pain and inflammation].

- *Dimethyl sulphoxide* [DMSO]. Solvent/liquid capable of dissolving things; easily penetrates the skin. It is a dangerous, unproven "remedy" for the pain and inflammation of arthritic affections.

- *Double-blind* [studies/trials]. A clinical trial in which neither the study staff nor the participants know which participants are receiving the experimental drug/substance and who are receiving a placebo or another therapy. Double-blind trials are thought to produce objective results, since the researchers' and volunteers' expectations about the experimental drug/substance do not affect the outcome.

- *Fibromyalgia.* A disorder [also known as fibromyositis, or tension myalgia] that primarily affects muscles and their attachments to bone. It does not cause joint deformity. Fibromyalgia is characterised by general muscle pain, stiffness, fatigue, sleeplessness, and numerous sensitive points at the sites where muscles join [to] the bones.

- *Genes.* Biologic units of heredity located at a specific position on a particular chromosome [cell structure composed of a linear thread of genetic material].

- *Glucosamine.* Glucosamine is found naturally in the body. It stimulates the formation and repair of articular cartilage.

- *Gout.* Inherited disorder [also known as crystalline arthritis] that is characterised by a variable level of uric acid [a normal by-product of foods] in the blood and sudden severe arthritis due to crystal deposits [sodium urate] within the joints.

- *Heberden's nodes.* Bony spurs that occur on the end joints of the fingers.

- *Hyaluronic acid.* Lubricating substance that is found in the normal joint fluid. Injectible hyaluronic acid is a FDA-approved treatment for osteoarthritis of the knee in the US.

- *Joint replacement.* Complete surgical removal of a painful joint, which is then exchanged for a man-made appliance.

- **Non-steroidal anti-inflammatory drugs** [NSAIDs]. Medications that are often used to relieve the symptoms of osteoarthritis. NSAIDs reduce the pain and swelling associated with inflammation. The most commonly used NSAIDs are aspirin, ibuprofen, and naproxen. NSAIDs are known to cause dangerous side-effects.

- *Osteoporosis.* Disorder in which bones and skeletal tissues become less dense and break easily. Osteoporosis occurs most often in post-menopausal women and elderly men.

- *Osteotomy.* The cutting of a bone. More specifically, an operation in which the surgeon divides the bone below the affected joint, and allows it to heal in a slightly altered position. The bone is realigned, with improved contact between the remaining healthy areas of cartilage in the joint.

- *Placebo.* A medically inactive substance that is used in controlled studies to determine the effectiveness of a test drug. Placebos have been shown to lessen symptoms in some people, most likely because of the individual's positive attitude about treatment.

- *Prostaglandins.* A group of substances that performs a variety of functions within the body, including control of inflammation and blood vessel permeability and regulation of hormones, stomach acid secretion, body temperature, and smooth muscle contraction.

- *Rheumatoid arthritis* [RA]. A disorder that is believed to result from an "auto-immune" process in which the body's immune system attacks itself. It is a system-wide disease that usually lasts for many years. In some patients, RA affects the heart, lungs, and eyes. Patients with active RA often feel feverish, or ill.

- *Spurs.* Osteoarthritic condition in which bony growths project outward from the ends of a bone in a joint.

- *Synovial fluid.* Thick, clear fluid produced by the synovial membrane, and found in joint cavities.

- *Synovial membrane.* Inner, smooth lining of the joint cavity.

- *Systemic lupus erythematosus* [SLE]. An inflammatory connective tissue disorder with variable features, including fever, fatigue, arthritis and joint pain, and red skin lesions on the face, neck and/or upper limbs.

- *Transcutaneous electrical nerve stimulation* [TENS]: A technique that directs small pulses of electricity to specific nerves. The aim is to reduce the sensitivity of nerve endings in the spinal cord, thereby closing the pain "gateways."

Index

NSAIDs [non-steroidal anti-
inflammatory drugs], 9
Nutraceuticals, 10, 117

Obesity, 18, 23
Oregon Health Sciences
University, 75
Osteoarthritis, 9, 15, 16, 19,
23, 27, 40, 93, 97, 108,
117, 118, 119
Osteophytes, 14

Piroxicam, 9
Primary osteoarthritis, 21
proteoglycans, 16, 17, 18, 22,
30, 33, 35, 38, 39, 45, 47,
48, 49, 56, 59, 64, 65, 76,
105

Quantum Magnetic
Resonance Therapy, 86

Sea cucumber, 71, 104
Secondary osteoarthritis, 21
Steroid injections, 83
Surgery, 85, 86
Synovial fluid, 13, 124

Therapeutic touch, 87
Traditional pain relievers, 82
Transcutaneous electrical
nerve stimulation, 87, 124
Turmeric, 72, 119

Vitamin C, 71, 73, 105

Yoga, 88

OTHER BOOKS IN THE NATURES HEALTH SECRETS
SERIES

NATURES HEALTH SECRETS
NATURE'S ASPIRIN
Rajgopal Nidamboor

*A PRACTICAL, UP-TO-THE-MINUTE BOOK ON ASPIRIN-
LIKE NATURAL HERBS TO COMBAT PAIN & ILLNESS*

Call it the "herbal aspirin" effect, or what you may, natural herbs
provide us a holistic medicinal tool-kit for optimal health and well-
being. They offer us the means to combat pain and other illnesses,
without the adverse side- or after-effects of traditional, or
conventional, non-steroidal anti-inflammatory drugs [NSAIDs].
This is not all. With the "demise" of the once-popular coxib drugs,
such as Vioxx, due to their deleterious effects on the heart, the
"climate," or need, for natural herbal remedies, to fill the gap, has
never been more pronounced. *Nature's Aspirin* explores what herbs,
in the form of simple but profound kitchen remedies, such as green
tea, ginger, turmeric, holy basil, rosemary etc., hold for us — a
mirror to the future of pain relief, including prevention and
treatment of a host of other disorders... such as cancer. Natural
herbs, it is rightly said, nurture our need for a safe and gentle
treatment plan, or option — without the side effects of
conventional medications.

ISBN 9781847161680

£9.99

NATURES HEALTH SECRETS
DETOX NATURALLY
Rajgopal Nidamboor

*A BOOK LIKE NO OTHER... EXPLAINS HOW NATURAL
DETOX CAN 'REV-UP' YOUR HEART
HEALTH & OPTIMAL
WELLBEING*

Ever thought of flushing out toxins from the body, or a non-surgical procedure that was safe, economical, and easy-to-use, to circumvent the need for bypass, or angioplasty? If you haven't, there's no need to search the horizons! For good measure, this natural, non-invasive therapy has proven benefits — based on actual patient results and studies conducted during the past five decades. Its name: chelation therapy. Chelation therapy is a simple form of treatment that not only reverses and slows down the progression of blockages in your heart, but also stalls the development of other age-related and degenerative diseases. Naturally.

There is also an additional benefit. The therapy improves symptoms associated with many other diseases affecting the body, though why this happens is not yet fully understood. Yet, the most important feature, which is also the most significant and verifiable aspect of the chelation treatment plan, is it happens... and, it also works.

ISBN 9781847161697

£9.99

NATURE'S HEALTH SECRETS
SEA MEDICINE CHEST
Rajgopal Nidamboor

*IMPROVING HEALTH THROUGH NATURAL SEA
REMEDIES*

Researchers suggest that the sea and ocean could become our new, big frontiers for deriving medicines in the 21st century. You name it — shark cartilage, shark liver oil, cod, or fish oils, mussel, sea cucumber, seaweed, oyster, shrimp, sponge etc., They are curative medicines. They are natural. They are available in profusion. Most importantly, they provide through their use a great degree of safety — for our optimal health and well-being, without the dangerous side-effects of conventional medications.

The best part — sea cure is risk-free and sure, so much so you will wonder why you have not tried some of its wholesome miracles yet! Not just a book, but a one-stop guide to expand on your health information-base — with the latest knowledge available on sea medicines — to lead healthy and vibrant lives.

ISBN 9781847161673

£9.99

Emerald Publishing
www.emeraldpublishing.co.uk

106 Ladysmith Road
Brighton BN2 4EG

Other titles in the Emerald Series:

Health (cont.)
Ultimate Nutrition Guide for Arthritis Sufferers
Finding Asperger Syndrome in the Family-A Book of Answers
Mental Health and the Community
Guide to Dementia care
Guide to Alternative Health and Alternative Remedies

Music
How to Survive and Succeed in the Music Industry

General
A Practical Guide to Obtaining Probate
A Practical Guide to Residential Conveyancing
The Property Investors Management Handbook
Writing The Perfect CV
Being a Professional Writer
Writing True Crime
Keeping Books and Accounts-A Small Business Guide
Business Start Up-A Guide for New Business
A Busy Managers Guide to Managing Staff
What Children Learn in the Classroom - A Parents Guide to
Primary Education

For details of the above titles published by Emerald, and how to
order, go to:

www.emeraldpublishing.co.uk